The Futı Yoga Therapy

Combining Science with the Sacred Roots of Yoga, Both in Personal Practice and as Integrative Medicine

A Collaboration

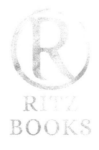

RITZ
BOOKS

The Future of Sacred Yoga Therapy: New Insights on the Impact of Yoga Therapy, Both in Personal Practice and as Integrative Medicine

Copyright © 2024 Steph Ritz
Paperback: 978-1-960460-23-3
Kindle: 978-1-960460-24-0

Curated and Published by RITZ BOOKS
Cover design, mandala, and interior layout by Steph Ritz
100% of this paperback's royalties are being donated to the non-profit: The International Association of Yoga Therapists. Kindle royalties from The Sacred Series support publishing BIPOC voices and minority-owned small businesses.

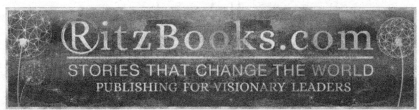

Table of Contents

Meet the Authors 4

Introduction 7
Nicole DeAvilla, E-RYT500, RPYT, RCYT, C-IAYT

A Guide to Longevity 17
Nicole DeAvilla, E-RYT500, RPYT, RCYT, C-IAYT

1 Million Healthy Happy Humans 27
Nicole DeAvilla, E-RYT500, RPYT, RCYT, C-IAYT

Yoga Therapy for Performance Anxiety:
Achieving Success through Self-Care and Mindful Practices.... 42
Ilene Cohen, MS, RDN, CLT, CDCES, C-IAYT

Harmony Unveiled:
Nurturing the Flame Through Ayurvedic Nutrition 60
Ilene Cohen, MS, RDN, CLT, CDCES, C-IAYT

Integrating Soul-in-Medicine with Your Yoga Therapy Path...... 78
Annie Kay, MS, RDN, E-RYT500, C-IAYT

A Military Yogi 96
Adhana McCarthy, MPAS, PA-C, C-IAYT

A Sherpa's Perspective of Yoga Therapy 112
Banton Dyer, CPT, C-IAYT

The Pain That Became a Separate Reality............................. 124
Nicole DeAvilla, E-RYT500, RPYT, RCYT, C-IAYT

The Lesson of the Smoke Detector.. 129
Nicole DeAvilla, E-RYT500, RPYT, RCYT, C-IAYT

Dharma and the Present.. 133
Nicole DeAvilla, E-RYT500, RPYT, RCYT, C-IAYT

The Digital Revolution in the Age of Energy......................... 145
Nicole DeAvilla, E-RYT500, RPYT, RCYT, C-IAYT

A Note from the Publisher.. 150
Steph Ritz with RitzBooks.com

Meet the Authors

The Future of Sacred Yoga Therapy looks at holistic health and wellness in your life and professional workplace, providing opportunities for you to educate and empower yourself with preventative approaches to improve physical, mental, and spiritual health.

The five Yoga Therapist authors in this collaboratively written book present expert guidance, stories of growth, and share their journeys into integrative healthcare through Yoga Therapy. They are also all certified by The International Association of Yoga Therapists (IAYT) – a non-profit organization that promotes ethical behavior on the part of Yoga Therapists, Yoga Therapy training programs, and organizations offers accreditations, research publications, and academic conferences.

These IAYT Certified Yoga Therapists seek to answer for you:
- What is Yoga Therapy?
- What are Yoga Therapy best practices?
- How can Yoga Therapy become a known term?

Nicole DeAvilla and Steph Ritz (publisher) met many years ago in a year-long marketing program, where Steph marketed for Nicole at the Symposium On Yoga Therapy And Research (SYTAR), which is one of the academic conferences hosted yearly by IAYT. In return, a few months later, Nicole taught Yoga Therapy and essential oils at Steph's redwoods writing retreat.

They've continued to work together ever since with Steph learning therapeutic yoga and Nicole receiving copywriting, photography, logo design, website design and more. Together they've written in Practice: Wisdom from the Downward Dog (along with co-author Banton) and in The Seed of Pure Potential.

Nicole and Steph have dedicated many hours to supporting IAYT. Nicole served on the first Accreditation Committee, the Meeting of Schools, has helped with fundraising and is a sponsor. Steph interviewed founding and key IAYT Certified Yoga Therapists as part of the non-profit's 30-year anniversary, and quotes from these interviews will be scattered throughout this book.

Ilene Cohen and Steph met the second time Steph attended SYTAR, and have been writing in the background together over the years. Ilene brings forward two chapters in this book, focusing on self-care practices to overcome anxiety and eating for body harmony.

Ilene brings passion and purpose to the fields of certified Yoga Therapy and nutrition. She has authored two peer reviewed publications, From Bliss to Balance: Using Yoga and Meditation in Diabetes Care" and Why Yoga: What Diabetes Educators Should Know in AADE in Practice, a Publication of the American Association of Diabetes Educators.

Specializing in mind-body integrative and functional medical nutrition therapy and therapeutic yoga, Ilene is known for her methodical critical thinking and supporting others to reach their highest potential.

Annie B Kay and Ilene are both Dieticians. While discussing this book project with Steph, they found they'd both been leading dandelion meditations. You'll find a calmness to the words in Annie's chapter.

Adhana McCarthy, a SYTAR keynote speaker, met at Steph's second SYTAR. When Adhana pulled one of Steph's Epic Story Prompt cards from prayer shaped ceramic hands, they stood rooted in place telling stories for what felt like 20 minutes while 400 people moved around them. Then the next day, Adhana came back to share another story with Steph. Here, she shares a non-stereotypical look at yoga, and the greater applications and implications of Yoga Therapy.

Banton Dyer met Nicole a decade ago at SYTAR. Steph met Banton when they all wrote together in another collaboration book a few years back. He credits his life to Yoga Therapy and pours his heart into being a sherpa for his Yoga Therapy clients.

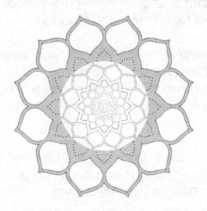

Yoga as a therapy is entirely different than regular yoga practice. The way we talk about every yoga practice is healing. It is a relaxation response. It is parasympathetic activation. Yoga Therapy is your adaptation of the yoga practice based on patients' or clients' physical or medical condition.

~Dillip, C-IAYT

Introduction
Nicole DeAvilla,
E-RYT500, RPYT, RCYT, C-IAYT

Ancient Wisdom Meets Modern Medicine at the Frontiers of Global Health

Though many people may be characterized by one extreme or another, such as either an introvert or an extrovert, a pragmatist or a dreamer and the like, rarely are they just that one thing without a trace of the other. Throughout my life I have found myself squarely in the middle of many of these dichotomies. I am equally an introvert and an extrovert, a pragmatist and a dreamer, a scientist and a metaphysicist and for me the list continues.

When I first learned through yoga that there are three doshas (you will learn more about this within this book) or constitutional types, I found myself trying to fit squarely into one of them. Later, when I had a proper reading by an Ayurvedic (the medical sister science to yoga) specialist, I was relieved to learn that I was nearly tri-doshic, equal parts of all three.

As I grew up I "learned" to separate many facets of my life. For example when I was at the Vanity Fair Social Club covering the Oscars as a social media correspondent, I didn't talk about how I could read or see the subtle energy of a person's chakras. I separated my scientist hat and my esoteric hat; my social butterfly was separate from my meditation lotus pad and so on. It wasn't until I began to spend time with Yoga Therapists that I felt that I could share more of myself in one setting. Among Yoga Therapists, science is as well respected as altered states of consciousness accompanied by euphoric states of bliss and connection to the divine.

I feel most at home when I can be and express all facets of myself. Yoga Therapy has allowed me to blossom in this way. This book expresses many of the facets of the lived experience of Yoga Therapists and their clients and the spiritual depths and rigorous science which surround and envelop it. This book is your invitation to explore Yoga Therapy on a personal level. It is also an invitation to a greater understanding of how Yoga Therapy can help many of the world's challenges and a glimpse of how organizations and institutions can benefit from investing in offering the preventive and healing benefits of Yoga Therapy to their people.

Where We Are Now

Imagine standing at the intersection of two worlds—ancient wisdom on one side, and modern science on the other. Each holds its own set of tools, philosophies, and possibilities. Now picture yourself, not just standing but thriving at this intersection, creating an unprecedented synthesis that could change the landscape of human potential. That's precisely where we are today, and the future couldn't be more promising.

At the moment with a world raging with war, devastating weather events, and a rising tide of lifestyle diseases, only a small number of people imagine seeing the future as promising.

Did you know that:

- Only 7% of Americans have optimal cardio-metabolic health?
- The number of people troubled by anxiety and depression continues to rise at alarming rates?
- Chronic pain is fast becoming a new global concern?
- Many family caregivers die before the person they care for because of the chronic stress associated with caregiving?

These are just a few bullet points in a sea of growing statistics. Yet these statistics represent real people. People who are dearly loved. People who are forgotten. People who might have lived a different life...

Millions and millions of people desperately need help.

You might ask — what new drugs do we need? Is there a new technology that can help? What can be done, if anything? How much will it cost?

The answer is simpler than you might expect. We already have the drugs and procedures required to cure many of the leading diseases that cause pain, suffering and premature death around the world but clearly it's not been enough. Do we need more of that or something else? We have that something else already. And it is very powerful. We have the time-tested practices and teachings of yoga and Yoga Therapy.

How can this be? Because Yoga Therapy addresses people in a holistic and lifestyle-oriented way. Yoga Therapists are uniquely trained and equipped to help people with lifestyle issues. Yoga Therapists are lifestyle experts. Many leading causes of death are lifestyle diseases. Without addressing lifestyle, we are only putting bandaids onto gaping wounds. When you combine modern healthcare with Yoga Therapy you get something powerful that has never been available before this point in time.

What is the Difference Between a Yoga Teacher and a Yoga Therapist? And Why Does it Matter?

My elevator answer is this: A yoga teacher needs a minimum of 200 hours of yoga teacher training. A Yoga Therapist needs to be an experienced yoga teacher and then needs an additional 800 hours (at a minimum) of specialized training. This additional training brings Yoga Therapists into the fold of integrative medicine.

While yoga itself is an extraordinary toolbox, nestled beside it, like two peas in a pod, is the practice and application of Yoga Therapy—a discipline designed to harness yoga's principles for therapeutic purposes. Tailored yoga practices can alleviate lifestyle diseases like obesity, diabetes, and hypertension, can address musculoskeletal, mental and emotional issues, and can help support patients during the treatment of illness and disease, such as cancer. The Yoga Therapist takes into account each individual's unique health needs, their situation and other healthcare resources they may or may not be receiving.

Yoga Therapy is not one-size-fits-all; it's the epitome of personalized medicine. Yoga Therapists are like skilled craftspeople who know which tool to use and when. They can delve into the physical postures, breathing techniques, meditation and mindfulness practices, philosophies and spiritual awareness to create a program that addresses the individual holistically. They might only use a simple breathing practice, a mantra or physical alignment to begin a healing journey with Yoga Therapy.

Yoga Therapists are also trained to work within a modern healthcare setting as part of an integrative medicine team. Some Yoga Therapists choose to work in their own private practice and rarely if ever interact with other health care professionals. However, they do know when and how to refer their clients to other health care professionals when the need arises for different or more extensive care.

As Yoga Therapists, we embrace both our traditional roots and teachings and science and the best of modern health care. A Yoga Therapist can seamlessly weave in spiritual support based on a person's background and preferences. This is one of Yoga Therapy's strengths: never imposing or assuming what will or will not give spiritual refuge and strength to an individual. Science shows that people who are connected to their faith tend to have better health outcomes. The Yoga Therapist is one of the few health care professionals trained to be sensitive and alert to a person's spiritual life or, conversely, respectful to that person's lack or indifference to the spiritual life.

Yoga Therapists bring to the table eons of practical experience and practices that not only can help save lives, can help to extend both the quality and length of life.

The Science

As I looked at the science and conducted research of my own, I was delighted to see how yoga fits right in with modern science, providing many of the elements of healthy living for a longer life. For example, yoga helps increase balance, grip strength, and leg strength, all factors which, when optimized, predict a longer life. Lack of the ability to balance, and lack of strength, predict a shorter life.

Yoga has also been shown to be effective at the cellular level, increasing telomere activity, for example. Here I will let one of many research studies speak for itself. Please note that "pranayama" refers to breathing exercises.

"Telomeres, the repetitive sequences that protect the ends of chromosomes, help to maintain genomic integrity and are of key importance to human health. Telomeres progressively shorten throughout life and a number of studies have shown shorter telomere length to be associated with lifestyle disorders. Previous studies also indicate that yoga and lifestyle-based intervention have a significant role on oxidative DNA damage and cellular aging."

"We explored the possible mechanisms of how asana, pranayama, and meditation might be affecting telomere length and telomerase. Moreover, results showed that asana and pranayama increase the oxygen flow to the cells and meditation reduces the stress level by modulating the hypothalamic–pituitary–adrenal axis. Summing up the result, it can be concluded that practice of asana, pranayama, and meditation can help to maintain genomic integrity and are of key importance to human health and lifestyle disorders."

Implication of Asana, Pranayama and Meditation on Telomere Stability by Mrithunjay Rathore and Jessy Abraham

One of the research studies I was involved in showed the positive effects of a yoga practice on respiratory health, and the respiratory, physical, and psychological benefits of breath-focused yoga for adults with severe traumatic brain injury (TBI): a PubMed research paper. Many people who survive their original injury will not die from their TBI, but rather from a respiratory illness. Thus, Yoga Therapy once again brings in an element of longer and happier life.

Chronic stress is one of the many challenges of today's modern world, and it doesn't look like it will get better anytime soon. The effectiveness of yoga in helping to alleviate and manage stress and its related disorders is well-documented.

In essence the work of a Yoga Therapist begins with relieving physical, mental, emotional and spiritual pain, trauma and imbalance. The Yoga Therapist's work helps people reach their highest potential. One's highest potential includes living the healthiest, happiest and longest life possible, as well as living life purposefully and spiritually.

A Beacon for Inclusion and Diversity, and a Quest for Peace and Calm

What makes Yoga Therapy so versatile is its universality. It transcends age, gender, ethnicity, and even physical capabilities. Yoga Therapy is uniquely positioned to encourage inclusion and celebrate diversity, by virtue of its adaptability and individual approach. This makes Yoga Therapy an ideal modality for addressing a variety of unique cultural and physiological needs, spreading its benefits across all strata of society.

The true beauty of Yoga Therapy lies in its universal applicability and its capacity to be highly personalized. The techniques and wisdom that helped alleviate my pain were the same that helped others, but each were selected and applied in a unique way. I've seen students quit smoking, regain joint mobility, and even find their smiles again. The stories are as varied as they are inspiring—

from those aging gracefully to others ready to embark on a journey toward longevity and holistic happiness.

This individual transformation creates a ripple effect that benefits not just the individual; his or her family or important relationships and the community at large are also benefited. Each personal victory becomes part of a collective experience that elevates the overall consciousness.

Now, more than ever, we find our world mired in turmoil, stress, and conflict. Yoga Therapy holds the key to rebalancing our inner lives and, by extension, fostering global peace. The meditative techniques employed by Yoga Therapists can teach us to remain centered amid chaos, and help us to reduce stress hormones, promote emotional equilibrium. Imagine applying this on a societal scale, where communities learn to manage collective stress, reducing societal divisions and promoting a culture of peace.

Conclusion

In the United States and elsewhere around the world, yoga has been commercialized and popularized and often reduced to physical exercise, with perhaps a touch of breathing and relaxation practices added for authenticity. Just as all forms of exercise are good for our health, and deep breathing and relaxation practices can calm our nervous system, this new offshoot of original yoga has its benefits.

Much of what is lost in these modern and trendy forms of yoga is retained in Yoga Therapy. Yoga Therapy preserves time-tested practices from the past and supplements those practices with the teachings of modern medicine. The future of Yoga Therapy is also the future of yoga. As the trends fade and new needs arise, one need only to look to the emerging field of Yoga Therapy to deal with those new needs.

Within the pages of this book, you will be given a glimpse, an insider's look, into the possibilities, the realities, the research, and the lives of real people, from diverse backgrounds who have been saved, helped or guided into transformative healing by Yoga Therapy, enriching their lives well beyond the healing process.

You will discover the power of a simple breath, the importance of yogic nutritional makeovers and what it means to be a Warrior Monk.

I can't wait for you to read and be inspired in the chapters written by my Yoga Therapist colleagues. Each one has their own inspiring journey. They are highly educated and trained, not only in Yoga Therapy but in other disciplines, including the fields of science, nutrition and the military. Their work has helped countless individuals.

We come together for this shared purpose: to spread the understanding of Yoga Therapy and how Yoga Therapy can help reverse the health and psychological burdens of our age. Truly, this sacred tradition has a future, and its future and success is inexorably tied to the future rise of global health and well- being.

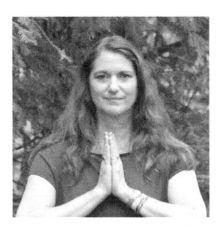

Nicole DeAvilla is a best-selling author, speaker, yoga educator, and coach with decades of experience. She is a well-respected Yoga Therapist and teacher at the Expanding Light Retreat Center, founded by Swami Kriyananda. Her book, *The 2 Minute Yoga Solution: FAST and EASY Stress and Back Pain Relief, for ANYONE at ANYTIME* highlights the benefits of yoga in a fast-paced modern life.

Nicole's passion for creating community, for connecting with people on an individual level, is born out in the programs she leads and her private client work. Her chakra readings are particularly helpful when you need guidance to unblock, unlock or discover either your next best small step or your next big leap! Want to be feeling free, abundant, supported and enjoying the waves of life? Let Nicole's insights joyfully guide you to connect with your inner spirit to help you reach your highest and most magnificent potential.

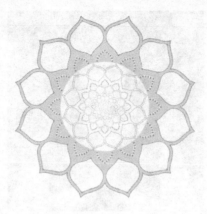

My goal from the beginning has been an integrative approach. I think the future of Yoga Therapy is integrative.

~Larry, C-IAYT

A Guide to Longevity
Nicole DeAvilla,
E-RYT500, RPYT, RCYT, C-IAYT

Let me take you back over 20 years to when I wrote my first best-selling book, "The 2 Minute Yoga Solution - FAST and EASY Stress and Back Pain Relief for ANYONE at ANYTIME". The following is the forward to that book, written before anti-aging, aging backwards and longevity science were popular on Instagram.

February 2012

The courtesy vehicle I was in began to swerve into the lane of oncoming traffic. Instead of looking at the road, the driver was looking at me and staring in disbelief. We had been chatting and my age came up—well, actually just the fact that I had a 16-year-old son (no, I was not a teenage mother). I felt lucky that there wasn't an oncoming car, which could have caused quite a bit of aging to both of us...

After learning my age, people often ask, "What's your secret?"

I answer, "Yoga."

"But hey," they say, "lots of people 'do' yoga and they all don't look this young—nor do they stay calm when they think they are about to be in a car crash. It must be your genes—but then genes can only take you so far, and they don't keep you calm—what IS your secret?"

"Yoga lifestyle," I answer. "I practice yoga 24/7." I go on to explain, to those who will listen, that yoga lifestyle is more than just practicing yoga postures at the gym. It's about a daily practice, lifestyle choices, and mental attitudes. The good news is that you don't need to set aside hours of time to get results, because you can incorporate yoga into all of your daily activities.

So what is the "yoga lifestyle?" Is it defined by the trendy yoga clothes that fashionistas now wear? The food we eat? Luxurious retreats and spas where yoga has become de rigueur? Hopefully (you may be thinking), it's not about grim austerities, denial, or giving up eating at restaurants. Rest assured that my secret is not about denial!

So is it the yoga pants that I wear almost daily? I admit that it is a great convenience and a bit of a perk nowadays that I can look "cool" when I come straight from work and pick up my daughter and her friends from school or dash off for a meeting with the school superintendent. No one even knows I came from work and that I was actually teaching yoga.

However, the only thing my daughter wanted last year for Christmas was a gift certificate to Lululemon's—for yoga pants. She does not practice yoga. She wanted them to wear to school like her friends do. I guess it's not my yoga pants that define my yoga lifestyle and are the secret of looking and feeling younger than my years.

Wearing cool looking clothes might get you in the mood—though, not necessarily for yoga. It's not a strict diet, though yes, I am a vegetarian and a healthy diet does make a difference. It's not practicing extreme yoga postures for hours a day—that will get you injured, not healthier.

For me, Yoga Lifestyle is about an attitude, a can-do spirit, and being realistic. Yoga Lifestyle is about all of the little things I do all day and the thoughts I think and the choices I make.

I practice affirmations. I take short yoga movement, breathing, and centering breaks throughout the day. I focus my mind at the pre-frontal lobes of my brain as often as I possibly can.

I practice the precepts of the Yoga Sutras—the most well-known is ahimsa (non-violence), which was made famous by Mahatma Ghandi. Whereas I am not trying to topple a government through peaceful means, I do try to act with loving kindness to others, as well as myself. That means no nasty thoughts about *my co-worker that just doesn't get it or no mental flogging myself for downing the brownie batter.*

Though I can sit for hours working on the computer or driving my two active children to opposite ends of the county for their activities, I do sit consciously in ways that raise my energy, rather than deplete it. I have learned how to take short movement and breathing breaks and how to keep my mind focused on moving forward and not stuck on the stress of how much needs to get done in so little time.

The great yoga master Paramhansa Yogananda explained that the minutes are more important than the hours, which are more important than the weeks, which are more important than the months, which are more important than the years. How true! We can have good intentions of living healthier, happier, more productive lives and then suddenly notice that a year or two or more have gone by and we still have that nagging back pain (in fact, it has probably gotten worse), we still seem to be spinning our wheels, and we still can't stop, focus, and be content and happy in the moment.

Techniques that I use daily are in this book. It only takes two minutes to change the way you feel now. When you feel better, you make better choices. When you make better choices, your physical and mental health improves.

With a busy lifestyle, it can be hard to carve out the time for a regular, traditional yoga practice—yoga pants or not. At other times, we can be so overwhelmed that we do nothing. With my private clients and yoga students, I feel that one of my most important jobs is to help them find ways to practice yoga daily, even if it is for just 2 minutes. This book gives you the tools and tips that I have been using for years for myself, my students, and clients.

Yoga works. But yoga works only if you practice it. You only need two minutes. What are you waiting for? Read on and start moving, breathing, and centering!

Fast forward to today. A fair question to me is – how's that anti-aging going for you now, 20+ years later?

As background, during these 20 plus years, I have had major abdominal surgery, and I re-injured my achilles tendon, aggravating an old injury that had initially required an operation in my high-school years and prompting a cascade of follow-on symptoms. Between the achilles pain, knee instability, and creeping hip and back pain, a little 2 Minute Yoga was all I could do. Add to that the stress of intense caregiving for more than one family member, of menopause that was not receptive to my 24/7 lifestyle, of maintaining a business, and of writing chapters in several books, I nevertheless said "yes" to a rigorous certification program about artificial intelligence. The result was that I was truly "running on empty. I guess I can't help being a pioneer: - I was one of the first yoga professionals to use social media in my business, was at the forefront of establishing national standards for the training of prenatal yoga teachers and international standards for the training of Yoga Therapists and was among the early wave of published researchers in the field of yoga research. The further result, of course, was that I got out of shape.

In addition to all that, for 40 years, my food and chemical sensitivities, and a tendency to sleep too little, have frequently produced inflammation throughout my body, especially in my joints and back where I have had past injuries. The inflammation spiraled fiercely out of control, resulting in frequent pain. So maybe you could say I was a mess.

My yoga practices kept me going and helped settle me down. Yoga reminded me to prioritize sleep, practice what I preach and devote more time to self-care. In addition to getting all the way back into my yoga practices - I added "smart supplements", including herbs, essential oils, vitamins and minerals, superfoods, and yes, the new rave, collagen, infused with some of the new "longevity" ingredients.

(https://nicole-deavilla.mykajabi.com/natural-solutions-to-live-longer-happier-with-spirit)

It really wasn't until a little over a year ago that I felt I was finally turning the corner - yoga, my new supplement routine, and basic yogic nutritional concepts such as cleanses and eating only "real" food, did the trick. So, when a year ago I was offered the opportunity to test my biological age and compare it to my calendar age, I was excited and a little nervous. I knew I wasn't going to get high marks, as I was still getting back into shape. I was actually relieved to learn that my biological age as measured by the Evolt BioScan, was exactly the same as my calendar age. I was told that was a really good sign!

A year went by. I am aware that I am still not back to my ideal level of health and wellbeing — caregiving, family responsibilities, running a business, enrolling in the AI program etc. have not been conducive to reaching those goals. So I told myself it was time for a check in, to see how I was aging. I was pleasantly surprised.

In fact, just this morning I was in a meeting with many of the students in my AI Mastery program. We were given an assignment to go into smaller Zoom groups and get to know each other, and to discuss what we do. Toward the end we had extra time and it came up that I had recently taken the biological age test again. I was happy to report that I did in fact "age backwards" by two whole years!

They were duly impressed until I told them how old I actually am. Luckily none of them were driving or else someone might have had a near accident like my driver over 20 years ago. When I told them that I am now 62 calendar years old and biologically 60 years old, they were floored. They thought I was much younger.

You see, the testing I took (and all of the similar biological aging tests of which I am aware), do not test for how youthful your skin, nails and hair look, nor measure the vitality that you exude and the energy or magnetism you feel and which is perceived by others. My fellow students and colleagues were picking up on these less easily quantified physical and energetic cues.

So was it the yoga or the supplements? Both. I can tell you that yoga is vital. By themselves, supplements won't keep you calm in a crisis, help you read other people's energy fields, develop your intuition, help you balance on one leg (an important predictor of longevity). But both together are very powerful.

So where is my Guide to Longevity you might be asking or demanding about now? I hope you see that longevity in my mind is about so much more than living longer. It is about living in the moment. Living a happier life with more energy and vitality. Living your dharma, your life purpose.

Your Guide to Longevity
The 8 Live. Longer. Happier. Pillars of Longevity

1. Move your body. Every day. Even if it's just 2 Minutes at a time. Incorporate balance poses, core strength, hand grip, and thigh strengthening yoga or other activities. Walk - get outdoors everyday if you can for the fresh air, and cardiovascular benefits.

2. Breathe. The practice of breathing helps in almost every area of your life. Science and experience back this up. It doesn't have to be fancy. Deep regular relaxed breathing is where you start.

3. Center. Centering is a powerful way to manage your stress. Managing your stress is helpful for living a longer life. Centering or meditation helps you focus, and helps grow otherwise shrinking gray matter in your brain, when done with yoga meditation techniques.

4. Community. In yoga we call it satsang. Be with others who lift you up, who care about you and want you to reach your highest potential. Spending time with others and socializing regularly is well documented to help increase lifespan.

5. A Diet that is healthy for you. When I say diet I am not saying that you need to lose weight. I am talking about a yogic diet that is mindful of your food sensitivities, your needs, your environment, and your resources, and is pleasant for you. Often it's what you don't eat that matters more than what and how much you do eat.

6. Smart Supplements. I say smart because there is a lot of junk out there that might actually be detrimental to your well-being. In our modern world, even if we buy only organic, and avoid processed foods, it is very difficult to get the full spectrum of nutritional components we need to thrive. The many stresses of modern life from air and water pollution to constant emotional stress inducing environments, require more heightened nutritional needs as does high performance whether physically and/or mentally.

7. Sleep. Getting good rest and sleep is about more than getting your beauty sleep. Just about every one of your biological systems is affected by the quality of your sleep. Sleep affects your brain health and function, as well as your immune, respiratory, cardiovascular, musculoskeletal systems and others. Lack of sleep encourages the stress response, inflammation, and other negative impacts to your mind and body.

8. Integrative Health Care. Do continue to get your regular checkups and follow the advice of your doctor. We are lucky to live in a time where we can get the best of both worlds — ancient teachings of yoga as applied to modern living coupled with life saving and enhancing advances in medical science. I have always liked as a guiding principle what Paramhansa Yogananda, my spiritual guide and guru, said in a book about self-healing through affirmations based on the science of yoga. He discussed how powerful thought is and how to use our mind for healing. However, he too was practical. He said if you break your arm and can heal it instantly by the power of your mind, do it. If not, doctors are very well trained in fixing your broken arm. Do let your doctor know that you are working with a Yoga Therapist and let them know that a Yoga Therapist has hundreds of hours of additional training in integrative health than a yoga teacher.

And don't smoke. Here is a story of how yoga can help with quitting smoking and other habits that shorten your lifespan or reduce your joy of life. Back when I was a fairly new yoga teacher, not the highly trained, experienced Yoga Therapist I am today, I had a student in my group yoga class at the YWCA, Union Square, San Francisco. She was quiet and shy. I barely knew her.

One day she came up to me after class and said she wanted to thank me for helping her to quit smoking. I was floored. I didn't know what to say, as I didn't even know she was a smoker. She went on to explain that after yoga class she would go home and smoke a cigarette. She noticed that the wonderful feeling she had from yoga class would disappear as soon as she smoked. So, she kept waiting longer and longer before having her cigarette to prolong the good feelings she had from her yoga class. Eventually, she went long enough that she was able to simply stop smoking altogether.

This is one dramatic example of how the simple practice of yoga helps people to more easily adopt other healthy lifestyle activities and habits. The National Health Interview Survey shows that practicing yoga helps people to adopt healthier lifestyles. On the one hand the simple practice of yoga helps people to adopt a healthier lifestyle. On the other hand, it may be more complicated or difficult to make these changes, and that is where a Yoga Therapist comes into the picture. They are lifestyle change experts and can help you make the changes you desire.

People come to Yoga Therapy because they hurt. They hurt physically, mentally, emotionally and/or spiritually. The science showing the effectiveness of yoga practices is what brings some people to a Yoga Therapist. Some come to Yoga Therapy because they have tried everything else and they are desperate to find some kind of relief. And they do find relief.

What keeps people returning to Yoga Therapy, after finding relief from their aches and discomforts, is the realization that they can go beyond relief to living a more calm, centered life full of greater vitality, focus and energy. And now, because of the recent discovery that yoga practices might be able to help prevent premature aging and other health conditions, more people and more organizations, such as business, non-profits, hospitals and the military, will be offering and counting on Yoga Therapy for prevention purposes.

The future may indeed bring more medical advances in treating and curing the ailments of old age. We are seeing that happening already. The future is also ripe for adopting the ancient, and now scientifically researched, practices of yoga. One does not need to be a millionaire trying all of the latest drugs and therapies to pursue a longer, healthier life. You can start for free right now - take six deep breaths and smile.

I do want you to know there are potential side effects of yoga practiced under the guidance of a qualified Yoga Therapist:

You might experience calmness in tense situations, greater health and vitality, glowing skin, and unexplained moments of joy and bliss. People may be more attracted to you in positive ways. They might even think you are younger than you look. You might get carded when buying alcohol at the store when you are in your 50's. Some people experience better focus, others feel new-found hope.

If you are experiencing any of these side effects, please tell both your Yoga Therapist and your medical doctor (because we do not replace your usual care of your doctor and health care team; we become part of your team), so they too can learn about these beneficial side effects and adjust your care accordingly, if at all.

The only group of people I encounter who are not surprised by my actual age are other Yoga Therapists. Many of them also look, act and feel younger than their age. We would love to have you come join us in feeling younger and happier.

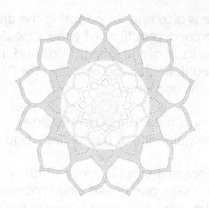

I see the future as finding common ground across all cultures where we can work together to build a global understanding and acceptance of Yoga Therapy in the world.

~Stephanie L., C-IAYT

1 Million Healthy Happy Humans
Nicole DeAvilla,
E-RYT500, RPYT, RCYT, C-IAYT

A Manifesto
What Keeps Me Up at Night?

What worries me and keeps me up at night? Well, nothing really. My yoga lifestyle practices work. If something were to keep me up at night it would be the following.

Fewer than 7% of people in the U.S. have optimal cardiometabolic health, with global rates of depression and anxiety climbing and disabling chronic pain exploding across our planet. We are in a health crisis.

By and large these diseases are "lifestyle" diseases. They are caused primarily by what we do and what we don't do in our daily lives.

Remember, if you incorporate the 8 Pillars of Longevity into your life, you will be protecting yourself from 7 of the top 10 causes of premature death in adults. If you ignore them, you are playing with fire.

Changing habits is not easy. Once you are on a downhill trajectory with lifestyle diseases, it can be even more difficult to make the changes necessary for a healthier, longer life.

Modern medicine has not been able to help people change their lifestyle. And so the numbers of individuals around the world who continue to suffer and die early continues to rise.

These are difficult problems, but there are solutions.

Even as a young child, I would worry about other people - the kid in my preschool who needed more love or a new doll, the child who was being shamed. It got to the point where my Mom would not watch the news if I was around because I would become too upset and want to help all the people in need. It didn't matter if it was the neighbor next door or a child in a different hemisphere; we had to do something right now!

Things haven't changed much. But my yoga practice has helped me to manage and channel my energy in concrete and productive ways. I focus on the things that I can change rather than dwell on what I have no control over. I have been inspired by the many people I have helped to have longer, happier lives over the 40 years of my yoga professional life.

I still want to help. To do more. Well, fortunately, we do have ways to solve the top causes of death that relate to lifestyle.

Yoga Professional Academy

The Yoga Professional Academy, which I founded, was born out of a desire to help more people, locally and globally, to eradicate unnecessary pain and suffering, to foster higher consciousness, and to help heal our planet and ourselves. It serves to mentor, educate, coach and support yoga professionals and yoga professional training directors and studio owners, while fostering a sense of community and belonging to those who are on the front lines of providing yogic services.

I could never do it alone. I am now using my 40 years of experience in the field of health and wellness to help mentor a new generation of yoga professionals, who will lead the way in the future. In doing this I have attracted the notice of other professionals, healers, entrepreneurs and authors who have asked me to help them reach out to and help more people. I say the more the merrier and healthier. And so I continue to serve.

I feel that at this point in my life, the best service that I can give is to train and support the new generation of Yoga Therapists and yoga teachers. They must be equipped with the knowledge, experience and business support they need to make a difference.

As a natural adjunct to this, I am supporting businesses, organizations, entrepreneurs, healers, authors, coaches and others aligned with similar values and aspirations through my newest programs and services, which go by the name Healthy, Happy Marketing – Grow Your Business Mindfully with Love.

Recently, I Realized This Is Not Enough.

I had big ideas about how to make a difference. It's easy for me to visualize a situation and see solutions clearly in my mind's eye. I can get inspired and tell other people about my ideas thinking they will get as inspired as I am. But in this case they weren't. I wasn't able to communicate properly.

As a Yoga Therapist I am aligned with the goal of finding and treating root problems rather than symptoms. I train my Yoga Therapist students and those I mentor to do that with their clients - look for the root causes and address them. Do not let an overly simplistic focus on symptoms get in the way of profound healing.

Something was getting in my way of creating profound change. So I stopped and went into the silence. I prayed. I meditated more often and longer. I had to practice patience. Before long people and experiences started coming to me.

I learned that if you want to make a difference, a real impact in the world, you need to tackle big problems and reach for the moon. I was challenged to dig deep and come up with audacious ideas. The bigger the problem it solves, the more magnetic your project becomes and the easier it is to attract top people to help you.

I dug deep. More meditating. More prayers. More stillness. It became clear, I needed to be more specific, more concrete and articulate a larger, more impactful vision. This is how the 1 Million Healthy Happy People Initiative was born. With this new found vision and articulation, people from diverse backgrounds and professions from around the globe react with enthusiasm and surprisingly often with offers to help!

Is This a Bold, Daring Initiative?
You bet! Buckle Up and Join Me on This Ride.

An army of Lifestyle Experts is needed to help the growing population from falling into the funnel of seemingly intractable lifestyle diseases, and to help to create positive meaningful, joyful lifestyle change instead. Who could fill this role? Yoga Therapists are experts on lifestyle — lifestyle medicine if you will.

The challenge here is three-fold. First, public and medical recognition of the benefits of Yoga Therapy as lifestyle medicine. Second, connecting those in need with a Yoga Therapist. Third, making sure we have ample numbers of Yoga Therapists ready to react to the call for help.

This initiative is designed to address all three challenges. At the heart of its mission is to connect those in need with a qualified Yoga Therapist. Through outreach, education, partnerships and publicity we aim to effectively communicate to the public why, where and how to find a Yoga Therapist and to help make it easy to make that connection.

In order to make these connections, the first challenge is tackling the lack of information and knowledge about the emerging field of Yoga Therapy. You might think of this as the publicity arm of the program. We intend to go much deeper and partner with organizations such as the International Association of Yoga Therapists and private companies with like-minded values, such as 360° Health Technologies. We seek sponsorship from compatible, value-driven businesses and institutions to support the monetary needs of the initiative. We also seek to support research on yoga interventions for lifestyle diseases.

Because Yoga Therapy is an emerging field, we need both to make people aware of its opportunities and potential global impact and to attract new talent to the profession. As part of this endeavor we seek to find ways to interact with and support the Yoga Therapist training programs and schools. In short, we seek to entice individuals into the field of Yoga Therapy.

Our Audacious Goal: Help 1 million people connect with a Yoga Therapist to get the education, guidance and support they need to either prevent or mitigate lifestyle diseases.

Let's Do a Data Dive! Apologies to those of you who are not data driven, it's me with my scientist hat! Feel free to skip if you like. I find these data driven statements a motivating call to action. Next we will get on to the business of yogic action taking.

- "At a global level, 7 of the 10 leading causes of deaths in 2019 were noncommunicable diseases."
  - ⇒ *The Top 10 Causes of Death* *https://www.who.int/news-room/fact-sheets/detail/the-top-10-causes-of-death*

- "In 2017-2018, only 6.8% (95% CI: 5.4%-8.1%) of U.S. adults had optimal cardiometabolic health..."
  - ⇒ *Trends and Disparities in Cardiometabolic Health Among U.S. Adults, 1999-2018* *https://www.jacc.org/doi/abs/10.1016/j.jacc.2022.04.046*

- "Globally, life expectancy has increased by more than 6 years between 2000 and 2019 – from 66.8 years in 2000 to 73.4 years in 2019."

- "... the increase in HALE [Healthy Life Expectancy] (5.4 years) has not kept pace with the increase in life expectancy (6.6 years)."
  - ⇒ *GHE: Life expectancy and healthy life expectancy* *https://www.who.int/data/gho/data/themes/mortality-and-global-health-estimates/ghe-life-expectancy-and-healthy-life-expectancy*

- "1.8 million annual deaths have been attributed to excess salt/sodium intake."
  - ⇒ *Global Burden of Disease Collaborative Network, Global Burden of Disease Study 2019 (GBD 2019) Results (2020, Institute for Health Metrics and Evaluation – IHME)* *https://vizhub.healthdata.org/gbd-results/*

- "In terms of attributable deaths, the leading metabolic risk factor globally is elevated blood pressure (to which 19% of global deaths are attributed), followed by raised blood glucose and overweight and obesity."

⇒   https://www.who.int/news-room/fact-sheets/detail/noncommunicable-diseases

- "1 in every 8 people in the world live with a mental disorder."

⇒   https://www.who.int/news-room/fact-sheets/detail/mental-disorders

- "In 2019, 301 million people were living with an anxiety disorder including 58 million children and adolescents."

- "In 2019, 280 million people were living with depression, including 23 million children and adolescents."

⇒   Institute of Health Metrics and Evaluation. Global Health Data Exchange (GHDx), (https://vizhub.healthdata.org/gbd-results/, accessed 14 May 2022)

- "Approximately 1.71 billion people have musculoskeletal conditions worldwide."
- "Musculoskeletal conditions are the leading contributor to disability worldwide, with low back pain being the single leading cause of disability in 160 countries."
- "Because of population growth and ageing, the number of people living with musculoskeletal conditions and associated functional limitations is rapidly increasing."

⇒   https://www.who.int/news-room/fact-sheets/detail/musculoskeletal-conditions

I look at this and want to jump up and down and shout "Look at what is happening! It's terrible! And we have the answers right here, right now, right in front of us! We can solve many of these big humanitarian problems!" But I don't do that - except occasionally at home. Because I practice yoga, I instead channel this energy into proactive steps. I am taking a big one now, writing this manifesto.

Change or Die

By all accounts the above numbers are not improving. I chose these particular examples because they all relate to NCD's noncommunicable diseases). In other words, for the most part, lifestyle diseases.

Research has shown that lifestyle interventions do in fact work — if people actually make those lifestyle changes. Most don't. Even when faced with the choice of living or imminent death, most fail to make the required lifestyle changes and die prematurely.

In some cases, poverty, and the lack of available resources and support can make change nearly impossible. However, note that in the United States fewer than 7% of Americans have optimal cardiometabolic health. Even when socioeconomic circumstances are not a barrier, most die rather than make lifestyle changes.

An article, by Alan Deutschman, published in 2007, called "Change or Die" highlighted both the problem and a solution. He cites research that shows that only 1 in 9 people make the necessary lifestyle adjustments when confronted with the choice. That means 9 out of 10 die prematurely from a preventable cause.

Believe me, I understand the difficulty of making lifestyle changes. Some of the changes I have had to make took some effort. Others I am still working on, trying to be consistent. My biggest and most stubborn lifestyle blunder? Not going to bed at regular times and sleeping long enough. So, I get it. I get the challenges. And I am well aware that I have been able to make as many lifestyle changes as I have because I have a regular yoga practice.

There Was One Big Exception

One famous program based on yoga and yogic principles was shown to increase a person's odds of successfully changing their lifestyle from 10% to 77%! This was not a one-off study with small numbers. This is the Dean Ornish program that has been studied and replicated and is now covered by Medicare. Through these lifestyle changes people are able to live healthier lives which help them to live longer.

So what is the difference? I won't go into all of the details here. I encourage you to read Deutschman's article and look at the work of Dean Ornish, who is also studying the effects of a yogic based lifestyle on cancer and Alzheimer's disease.

Here is a quote from the article:

> "Even when leaders have reframed the issues brilliantly, it's still vital to give people the multifaceted support they need. That's a big reason why 90% of heart patients can't change their lifestyles but 77% of Ornish's patients could -- because he buttressed them with weekly support groups with other patients, as well as attention from dieticians, psychologists, nurses, and yoga and meditation instructors."

An integrated approach with yoga and meditation instructors - the forerunners of Yoga Therapy - was able to make unheard of results. Yoga Therapists are uniquely trained to help problem solve on an individual level, deliver personalized science based solutions and deliver the support and encouragement that is part of this recipe.

Are you doing a double take about now? Can people really live a longer life through lifestyle changes? There is a growing body of evidence and consensus that lifestyle changes really do positively affect lifespan and healthspan. Here is Dr. Wong of Kaiser Permanente on the topic of a plant-based diet for example:

"A plant-based diet is associated with a longer and healthier life span," said Dr. Wong. "It can help prevent chronic conditions such as heart disease, obesity, and type 2 diabetes. There's also a lower overall risk of cancer — especially colorectal cancer."

Just think what qualified Yoga Therapists (who teach many modalities of yoga, including breathing, meditation and more) can do in the realm of prevention and participating as a valuable member of an integrated healthcare team.

This knowledge is not new. Why is it not more widespread? Why aren't more people being helped to change their lifestyle, with yoga being a top recommendation? There are many reasons - social, economic, and political. These barriers can be overcome.

We Are Moving Forward

Ever since the first "Symposium of Yoga Therapy and Research" in 2007, my Yoga Therapist colleagues and I have been excited and thrilled to see the emerging field of Yoga Therapy move from its infancy to where it is today. I recall with some embarrassment the presentation of my first poster research presentation I presented at this SYTAR - basically, unsophisticated poster flyers. However, what I remember most is conversations with medical doctors, the TV star of "Yoga with Lillian" and people from around the world who were as excited as I was to learn more, do more and help more.

The evidence of yoga's role in helping people manage stress is convincing, and very promising. The U.S. military has invested in research and programs in yoga for veterans with PTSD, chronic pain and other conditions.

I attended the very first IAYT, Symposium of Yoga Research, SYR, in 2010. Since then, I have noticed that yoga research is playing a larger role in academic institutions.

At SYR there are often representatives from the National Institution of Health (NIH) attending and encouraging yoga research. They see what isn't working in healthcare and they see the potential for yoga to fill in the gaps.

Including more yoga research is now part of the National Center of Complementary and Integrative Health, NCCIH's strategic plan.

The NIH now has an eBook, for patient use that covers the reasons on why to try yoga, what the science says and how to start safely.

In other words large institutes are now beginning to see the benefits of yoga as therapy.

Even though I am a yogi, I like to move fast. I love seeing these changes, both in institutions and in individuals. Back when I opened one of the first yoga studios in San Francisco, no one understood what I was talking about at networking events when I would say I run a yoga studio.

"What? You have a yogurt shop?" they would quizzically ask. It was in the 1980's when the first soft frozen yogurt shops were opening and were all the rage.

Much progress has been made. Still only a small portion of the population has benefited by or has access to the healing benefits of yoga.

Like many, I wish these changes could happen faster.

We can move forward. We can make a difference. I implore you to do your part, even if it's just being a cheerleader for the cause, or join to support our team to help save lives, to help improve quality of life, and to save money through healthcare cost savings.

I Was a Thorn in Their Side

I was named to the first International Association of Yoga Therapists (IAYT), Accreditation Committee, which was charged with implementing the newly-adopted standards for the minimum training of Yoga Therapists and the rules and methods for Yoga Therapy schools to apply for accreditation. While serving on the Committee, I often bugged my fellow committee members and the then Executive Director of IAYT. My mantra was, "None of this matters if we don't have good jobs for Yoga Therapists."

The great need for Yoga Therapists was clear in our minds. By then even top military brass were convinced that yoga worked and they wanted to hire more Yoga Therapists. Their request for certification or some sort of standards to identify qualified Yoga Therapists was one of the motivating factors for IAYT to work as quickly as possible to put in place accreditation and certification standards. In essence it's a marketing job to bring awareness to those who make decisions, those who hire and those who are in need. To IAYT's credit they have helped elevate the field of Yoga Therapy and make it a more well known and respected field in integrative medicine.

Did I tell you my mom says I was always impatient? – I probably was a thorn in my mom's side too! Though my yoga practices more or less keep me "Even minded and cheerful at all times" - a saying of Yogananda's - , I still care deeply about needless suffering in the world. Let's help people now!

First, I supported and wrote some of my own peer reviewed pub-med research on yoga. I taught therapeutic yoga before Yoga Therapy was official. I helped launch Yoga Therapy training schools. I continue to be a faculty member for Ananda's Yoga Therapist Training and other programs. I offer coaching and group continuing education programs for yoga professionals. I have been wearing my policy wonk hat, my researchers hat, my yoga professional faculty, coach and trainer hat, and my esoteric read-your-chakras hat. Now I feel the need to get out my marketer hat to help the cause.

I've always been an entrepreneur, so I am framing the next step as a marketing challenge to create a vehicle for all who want to jump on board. The goal is to connect 1 million people to a Yoga Therapist. I am ready to step on the gas! Don't worry though, because of my yoga, I will drive safely!

So How Does the 1 Million Healthy Happy Humans Initiative Work?

There is ample evidence that Yoga Therapy can make a meaningful impact on changing people's lives through lifestyle and other yogic interventions, such as meditation, breathing practices and physical postures.

The problem is that little is known and understood about Yoga Therapy, because it is an emerging field. This project aims to change that. We want to:

- Make the health benefits of yoga and Yoga Therapy more well known in health care and medical settings.
- Make the health benefits of yoga and Yoga Therapy more

well known to the general population.

- Provide guidance on how and why to select a Yoga Therapist.
- Shine a spotlight on the field of Yoga Therapy and Yoga Therapists.
- Create more interest in the field and attract more students to study and become Yoga Therapists.
- Educate and create collaborative partnerships with the medical field.
- Support and collaborate with IAYT.
- Foster new and continuing research to bolster the efforts to bring Yoga Therapy to more people.
- Build strong relationships with businesses and organizations to help fund the program.

We are already finalizing talks with our first sponsor, who will provide us with the necessary technical platform to monitor and track progress and create data for research. Thanks to all of the scientists, marketers, organizations and individuals who have cheered us on as well as made valuable contributions to this cause. This includes the many Yoga Therapists who have already said "yes", they are ready! Bring it on!

How We Plan to Track 1 Million Happy Healthy Humans

Yoga Therapists opt into the 1 Million Happy Healthy Humans Initiative via an app-based platform. Every month they will log in and report the number of new Yoga Therapy clients they have. We will collect some basic information from the Yoga Therapist such as:

- Years practicing as a Yoga Therapist
- Average number of clients seen monthly
- Place of education
- Specialties, if any

Clients will remain anonymous. No identifying information on individual clients will be collected.

The following data is expected to be collected:

- Demographics; gender, age, location (by zip or country codes)
- Types of issues for which people go to see Yoga Therapists, such as respiratory, musculoskeletal, cardio,
- Severity of issue

At this time, no follow-up will be conducted.

From this, we will know when we reach 1 Million new Yoga Therapy clients. The data derived from this project will be presented in scientific studies and/or surveys that will inform us about the nature of Yoga Therapy use and application. We aim to create publicity around this cause, and to create a collaborative community of fellowship.

We Are Confident When Lifestyle Diseases Meet Lifestyle Experts, it's the 1 Million Healthy, Happy Humans Who Win

The National Center for Complementary and Integrative Health has clinical guidelines, scientific literature and information for both medical professionals and patients on the health benefits, tips, and the state of the current research on yoga. They look at over 30 categories of yoga for health.

These are the sources from the NCCIH Clinical Digest for Health Professionals and Yoga What You Need to Know. You can read the details and get the complete list of references here:

https://www.nccih.nih.gov/health/providers/digest/yoga-for-health-science

https://www.nccih.nih.gov/health/yoga-what-you-need-to-know

Yoga is considered a safe practice when done under the supervision of a qualified yoga teacher or yoga therapist, and with permission from one's doctor if under medical care. Yoga and Yoga Therapy can be made accessible and inclusive at low cost for diverse populations with a wide range of socio-economic statuses and locations.

Additionally, people like yoga! Advances in technology and increasing personal and institutional awareness of the benefits of yoga is breaking down barriers to access already.

Any new scientific discovery takes time to go from, "This is proven. We know it works," to have doctors, be educated and for them to change their habits and implement it in their care and for the public to be aware and open-minded enough to want to try something new or seek it themselves.

They often say that, with any scientific research, it can take at least 10 years before it gets put into practice on a large scale. We're moving at breakneck speed in terms of this being accepted by the public and in health care settings and used more. There is more familiarity, more use of yoga and Yoga Therapy for better health and wellness. In the big picture, the use of yoga for health in modern settings is expanding quickly. But is it fast enough for the people suffering today?

In conclusion:

There is a great need.
There is much work to be done.
There is great enthusiasm to do this great work.
There are many people ready to help.
Let's get started!

How do you want to help?

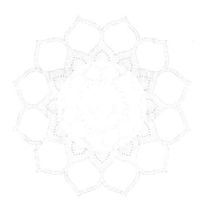

I think it's very important, both from a Western and Eastern perspective, that yoga is viewed as an important adjunctive intervention that can complement normal medical procedures and go to places where Western medicine has not yet been able to understand.

~Richard, C-IAYT

Yoga Therapy for Performance Anxiety: Achieving Success through Self-Care and Mindful Practices

Ilene Cohen, MS, RDN, CLT, CDCES, C-IAYT

Embark on a transformative exploration of Yoga Therapy's remarkable capacity to alleviate the debilitating grip of performance anxiety.

This chapter serves as a guiding light, illuminating the profound nexus between the relentless pressures of performance and the profound healing potential of yoga. Delve into the intricate tapestry of yogic practices and philosophies, discovering how this ancient tradition serves as a powerful conduit for emotional well-being amidst the chaos of modern life.

Advocating for the indispensable role of self-care in achieving enduring success, we delve into the transformative power of nurturing the self through compassionate practices. Journey through the realms of stress-reduction, where breath becomes the steadfast anchor amidst turbulence and meditation emerges as a potent elixir, enhancing cognitive fortitude in the face of adversity.

With each conscious breath, with each moment of stillness cultivated, transcend the paralyzing grip of fear and embark on a deeply personal odyssey toward self-discovery and empowerment. Through the timeless wisdom of yoga practices, spread your wings, soar beyond limitations, and reclaim the spotlight of your own existence with unwavering grace and resilience.

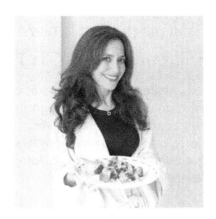

Ilene Cohen is a nationally recognized Registered Dietitian Nutritionist, IAYT-Certified Yoga Therapist, Ayurvedic coach, Certified LEAP Therapist, and Certified Diabetes Care and Education Specialist.

As an author, speaker, and coach, Ilene leads a thriving virtual group private practice, PranaSpirit Nutrition & Wellness, LLC dba Ayurvedic Path to Wellness™ and is also the owner and founder of RefreshExams, LLC, providing expert dietitian board exam preparation.

Since 2015, Ilene has helped hundreds of people transform their lives with stress-reducing breathing and meditation techniques, and performance and test-taking anxiety strategies.

Using her in-depth insights and intuitive nature, she specializes in combining her unique background as a dietitian and Yoga Therapist to harness self-care strategies for greater success in your life. Some of her go-to tools include meal planning, Ayurvedic Dosha assessments, and Myers Briggs evaluations for decreasing performance anxiety and building confidence.

https://www.liinks.co/ilene.cohen

Bridging the Gap Between
Performance Anxiety and Yoga Therapy

In the realm of various professions, the pursuit of success often goes hand in hand with an unwelcome companion—performance anxiety. The pressure to excel in board certifications, to deliver impactful presentations, or even to navigate significant career transitions can trigger overwhelming stress, leaving us feeling like we're standing at the edge of an abyss.

My journey into the world of Yoga Therapy wasn't just about personal wellness; it was an exploration of the profound connection between the mind and body, and how yoga can be harnessed as a powerful tool to combat performance anxiety. It was this revelation that led me to develop strategies, drawing from my own experiences and extensive knowledge in dietetics, to help my students prepare for their dietetics board exams while managing their test anxiety.

But my voyage didn't end there. As an avid yoga practitioner, I encountered my own moment of truth during my 500-hour yoga teacher training, an experience that bore an uncanny resemblance to the performance anxiety my students grappled with. It was a reminder that even the most well-prepared individuals can falter under the weight of stress. If I could turn back time, there's something I would do differently, and that is to incorporate meditation, pranayama (breathing techniques), and yoga nidra into my preparation regimen. These practices can significantly reduce performance anxiety and elevate one's chances of success.

Join me on this journey as we delve into the holistic approach of Yoga Therapy, exploring how it can be a transformative force in managing performance anxiety, from students preparing for dietetics board exams, to live videos, interviews and teaching auditions, and to anyone standing on the precipice of a significant challenge.

Breathing Through the Fear:
A Journey from Stage Fright to Speaker Spotlight

Okay, let me tell you a story. This is about my grad school days and, well, performance anxiety. Back then, presentations were a rarity for me, and my fear of stage fright was intense. There's this one time I had to get up in front of the room. I hadn't done many presentations in grad school, and my track record in college wasn't much different. The fear of stage fright was real.

So, I stood up, ready to speak, and the next thing I knew, I was on the floor. I had hyperventilated. I could hear my professor asking if I was okay, the whole class looking at me, unsure if I was going to be alright. It was a tough experience, a vivid encounter with performance anxiety.

This was before I discovered yoga, before I knew the power of self-care, especially when it came to breathing. That incident illustrates what performance anxiety feels like without the tools to navigate it.

Fast forward to my yoga teacher training. I had some tools, but the anxiety lingered. It wasn't as bad as hyperventilating, at least I could breathe, but it still wasn't a walk in the park.

Now, here's the twist. When I got up in front of the room again, armed with the tools I gained from yoga, things were different. I presented my material confidently. My teacher asked if I was sure I could do it. Without hesitation, I said yes. And I did it.

Now, cut to the present. I'm a national speaker. I've presented at the Food & Nutrition Conference & Expo. I've spoken at conferences all over the country, locally and nationally. I've hosted numerous webinars, and guess what? I enjoy it. No longer do I get that overwhelming nervousness before I speak.

The journey from being paralyzed by performance anxiety to confidently addressing a national audience has been transformative. Yoga became my anchor. Deep breathing, meditation, and other techniques became my allies. Embracing these tools didn't just mitigate performance anxiety; it made me a better speaker, a more effective presenter.

This journey is a testament to the profound impact yoga can have on performance anxiety. From the trembling fear on the floor to confidently commanding a stage, the evolution is real. Yoga didn't just equip me to deal with performance anxiety; it empowered me to conquer it, turning what was once a crippling fear into a source of strength. It's a journey that speaks to the transformative power of yoga in overcoming obstacles and becoming the best version of ourselves.

My Discovery of Yoga

After spending almost a decade working as a clinical dietitian in hospitals, outpatient clinics and diabetes centers, I got recruited by a disease management company in Texas for my ability to speak Spanish fluently and serve a large Hispanic population in a union. The pay was incredible and I received an increase in my salary by over 35 thousand dollars per year plus a sign-on bonus! I maxed out my 401K, went for Ayurvedic massages (which I still get less periodically, but they're an important part of my daily self-care) every two weeks and was living life.

But then I started getting burned out; I was working over 80-hour weeks and I felt like my health was on the line. Fortunately, I had been practicing yoga for the past year, which I know saved me. To spare my health, I ended up quitting my full time job, taking the money and signing up for a 30-day 200-hour yoga teacher training course.

That gave me one month to escape, but also to soul-search. It was all about self-care. I would say that the greatest lesson I've learned in the process has been the importance of self-care.

Self-care for me was practicing yoga, but most importantly, it was the benefit I got from it - improved breathing, freedom, stress reduction, improved sleep and eating habits. As a driven, dynamic go-getter, I was prone to burnout, so this also really helped nurture that aspect of myself to refuel the well. I even dropped in weight and became too thin. (I'm one of those high metabolism people who burns everything under stress so it really helped salvage me.) I learned to stay present and take things at a slower pace. As all of the students in the teacher training program went around the circle, I heard repeatedly, "I'm here because I left a stressful corporate job!" and I was included in that choir, since I left a job in the disease management company where I was working 80 hours per week (a story for another book). I was working for this company and working too hard. I went to the yoga teacher training because I had to quit my job as it was hurting my health. So, while I remained a dietitian, I pulled the yoga piece into it, which became part of my career in the same way dietetics did, as a result of personal experience.

Before I dive into the crux of this chapter- the techniques I'll help you employ to manage performance anxiety and achieve success- something happened to me in my 500-hour advanced yoga teacher training that shifted things for me and taught me a valuable lesson that I can bring to my students.

Why am I telling you this story? Failing happens to the best of us, even if we know what we're supposed to do.

So even for me, it's beneficial to have this chapter as a tool guide to come back to over and over again. Even though I know better, I still managed to fail. So, stop beating yourself up; let's put the tools in motion and move on. Many of my students have failed their exams anywhere from one to several times. Never give up.

Day of the Exam

It was time for our midpoint practical teaching exam. I prepared so much for my yoga teaching sequence, practicing it daily to the point I was singing my cues in the shower. Many of you may not know what happens in a yoga training, but simply put, each student teacher gets the chance to stand up in front of the group and teach their sequence, as if they're teaching a class. I didn't sleep at all the night before the exam. I went and booked a hair appointment to give me confidence and was on an adrenaline rush.

My turn came. I got up in front of my entire class and all my teachers were staring at me with the pens and papers. (Yes, yoga can be stressful when you're being tested!) I got up on the stage area and started teaching. All of a sudden, my mind went blank. I couldn't remember my sequence! I stopped and said to my audience, "I can't do this." My teachers said, "Just do your best. Don't be so hard on yourself." Well, I didn't exactly pass this exam. I failed my yoga teacher training practical mid-point exam.

I could have wallowed in misery but, instead, I told myself, "Ilene, you're a great teacher and you can do it!" The next day, I volunteered to get up in front of the room and teach a sequence. I got up and taught an amazing sequence. My teacher met with me after and said, "Wow, what a change from yesterday. I wasn't going to give you a class on the schedule after the exam yesterday, but I will add you to the schedule in the next couple of months."

Victory! I learned that the strength I get from failing is stronger than I would have gotten had I not failed that time. No matter how stressful and embarrassing this experience was, I didn't only succeed in the end, I excelled. You can, too. Many first time test takers have come to me feeling nervous and/or anxious that they were going to fail. So whether you're a first time test-taker or repeat tester, or are giving your first speaking engagement or audition, there's always the fear of the unknown. I hope this instills you with more confidence to persevere, no matter where you are in the journey!

Self-Care Strategies for Greater Success in Your Life

Before I tell you my next story, I just want to encourage you, whether you practice yoga or not, to know what I'm going to teach you will not be hard. There won't be any need for strength or flexibility - there are modifications to these couple of poses and if you're inspired to jump into one of my online yoga classes that's great. Breathing is KEY. One of the things I hear from my students is that they start hyperventilating and I know that stress makes people forget to breathe! My most successful clients said they practiced the breathing techniques I guided them on every night and before and during their exams. In this chapter we're going to talk about mindset - which is part of yoga, too.

I became a yoga teacher in 2007 and, honestly, my story in a nutshell is that I was not taking good care of myself and yoga saved me. I was working in my first job after my dietetic internship and, despite my colleagues leaving on time, I stayed until 7-7:30 pm every night to see my patients and get my work done. I would get home too late to wind down, end up going to bed late and then I was up early again for work. In hindsight, I was much better as an outpatient RD because I liked to take my time to educate and counsel my patients and inpatient wasn't much of a setting for that. nonetheless, I needed a different outlet to stop me from working too hard.

I remember sitting at lunch with one of my dietitian co-workers who suggested to me to try yoga. It was so random. I remember my response to her was, "Yoga? Isn't that about breathing?" The receptive one I am led me to try a kundalini yoga class at my gym. I loved it so much, it became an every Sunday early evening outing for myself. I loved the teacher and practice. I decided to take it a step further and try a yoga class at a yoga studio. When I walked into the yoga studio, where I ended up doing my teacher training, I remember the calm vibe, the smell of essential oils, the warm way everyone greeted me - this was in the middle of NYC where things were so fast-paced. I felt like it was a great escape for me. I started attending yoga classes there three times per week, including my weekly restorative yoga class.

Restorative yoga is a grounding and calm practice where your body rests on props, bolsters, blankets, etc. For those of you who haven't tried it, it feels like you're lying in bed on top of a super comfortable mattress with pillows supporting your body. I taught my students in our group program a class on power yoga poses to build confidence. My students loved it, both first-timers and those who have practiced before. I was inspired by Amy Cuddy's Ted Talk on "Power Poses." Her research is impressive: job interviews were significantly more successful when subjects stood in positions where they were open - meaning, arms wide, legs and arms uncrossed.

I knew that my goal was to teach my students how to stand in an open way that improved their posture and made them feel stronger.

My favorite confidence building yoga poses included in my sequence were:

- Tree pose with arms wide overhead

- Warrior 2 pose

- Low lunge with arms overhead

- Tadasana (standing mountain pose)

- Gate pose

Disclaimer - Before beginning a yoga practice or any of the practices in this book, you acknowledge that it is your responsibility to ensure that you are participating in a safe environment. If you suspect that you may have an ailment or illness that may require medical attention, you understand that you should consult with a licensed physician without delay.

Yoga has always been my anchor for every struggle I've been through in my life and career. I want to share three of my favorite yoga poses that create confidence.

Warrior 1 and Warrior 2 (Virabhadrasana 1 and Virabhadrasana 2) - elements and benefits: power, confidence, grounding. Elements of power and expansiveness.

Tree pose - elements and benefits: balance, confidence, posture, growth, calm focus

As one of my students said:

"Since I've started yoga with Ilene Cohen on Fridays, it's actually helped me relax!!"

"I'm excited for the breathing techniques scripts! And, the breathing/yoga are a great addition to the studying plan!"

When the going gets tough, just breathe

When I asked my yoga teachers what advice they had for me heading into my 200-hour yoga teacher training final practical exam, they both looked at me and said simultaneously, "Breathe." It sounds so simple. Breathing is something we humans do automatically, but then why is it so hard for us to remember to do it?

When confronted with a stressful situation, the '"fight or flight" response takes over - which means that our cortisol levels rise, blood flow moves away from our central organs into our hands and feet, preparing us to "run" from a perceived threat. Can you believe that taking an exam can cause this reaction in your body? So, we have to remind ourselves to breathe. But it works and that's why I'm passionate about teaching yoga breathing techniques to my students to manage test anxiety and/or build confidence. And I'm just as passionate about helping people to manage performance anxiety through yoga and Ayurveda.

I'm going to guide you in a breathing technique that I give my private students before their exams. I made a special bonus audio recording of this breathing technique so you can play it each day, headed to your exam, whenever you need it. Here's more from a client about our breathing techniques and the scripts you're about to learn:

"Ilene, when I get stressed at work I practice your breathing and

it helps me!! I stop and take breaths."

"Before I would just get really mad and stay that way all day!"

"It sounds silly, but just the little things help out!!"

"Ilene, thank you for sharing with us!!"

And for my client, the breathing helps her stay present and improve focus for her studying.

The breathing definitely helps me as well.

I'm doing the carb-counting practice and breathing through it as we speak.

I can't wait to support you on your journey into how yoga can help you with the stress management you need, including breathing and meditation.

2-minute performance success breathing/meditation

I love to start out by encouraging my students to think of a mantra. A mantra is a word or short phrase that can bring you into a place that feels good, that enables you to accept yourself as you are in whatever situation you're in. Here are a few mantras I've given to my students. Think of a special short phrase - around 3 words - that feels good to you. I'll give you a few to get you started. Try one or more of these to see which you like best or try making one of your own:

- I am successful.
- I am whole.
- I deserve success.
- I am confident.
- I am strong.

Close your eyes. Find a comfortable place where you can relax for the next two minutes.

Bring your awareness to your breath. Notice the air going in and out of your nostrils. If you're lying down or are seated, you can place your palms on your abdomen.

Notice the rise and fall of your belly, like a balloon. Notice the inhale. Is the air warm or cool?

Now on the inhale, imagine your mantra in your mind's eye. Maybe you hear yourself saying the mantra to yourself.

Breathe in the success, the positive, and what you want to embrace.

On the exhale, as you let the air go, like you're deflating a balloon, let go of anything you don't need. Let go of stress. Let go of judgment. Let go of failure.

Your inhale infuses you with strength, confidence, and fulfillment. Your exhale gets rid of anything that doesn't serve you right now.

Repeat this process on each round of breathing for 2 minutes or more. See, it wasn't hard, right? When you commit to just two minutes, it becomes doable. Then you can increase if you want. The most important thing is to be consistent. This is something I practice in my own life. It leads to a great sense of accomplishment when you know you're moving forward.

My Three favorite stress-reducing breathing techniques

1. *Alternate nostril breathing (Nadi Shodhana Pranayama)*

2. *Three-Part Breath (Dirgha Pranayama)*

3. *Buzzing Bee (Brahmuri Pranayama)*

If you're sold on my story and ready to try some breathing

strategies, you'll love (I hope) my favorite three. These breathing techniques bring me back to my yoga teacher training days. The good news is, they're all relatively easy to do, you don't need any special equipment to do them, and their rewards in terms of reducing performance anxiety are worth their weight in gold.

Breathing technique #1:
Alternate nostril breathing (Nadi shodhana pranayama)

The purpose of this technique is to create balance. It balances the left and right sides of the brain. The easiest way for me to remember the differences is that the right side is the more creative side and the left side is the more analytical side. So not only will it relax you, it will balance out the two sides of your brain that you need for the exam. You might think you need only the analytical side of your brain, but consider this: when you have an upcoming performance where you have to act in a certain role, whether it's giving a keynote presentation, a Tedx talk (if you're lucky enough to get on the big stage), an audition, or another performance, a little imagination can really help!

1. Start by placing your thumb around your right nostril and ring finger around your left.

2. Lift your thumb and inhale into the right nostril.

3. Close and block both nostrils ** If you are pregnant, do not block both nostrils. Continue to breathe freely throughout.

4. Lift your ring finger and exhale out the left nostril.

5. Repeat the process for 6 rounds.

Breathing Technique #2:
Three-Part Breath

What I love about this breathing technique is the rhythm and focus on the exhalation. Think of your inhalation as the more energizing breath and your exhalation as the more calming breath. While you need to balance your energy, when you're trying to calm yourself down, it can be a total lifesaver. It also helps improve focus because you're inhaling in three parts.

1. Inhale one third of the way into the belly.

2. Inhale another third of the way into your lower rib cage.

3. Inhale the last third of the way into your upper chest.

4. Pause at the top of the inhale, then slowly start to exhale out.

5. Make your exhale last as long as you can stretch it, without strain.

Breathing Technique #3:
Brahmuri (Buzzing Bee)

When I learned this during a 300-hour yoga teacher training, it became an immediate favorite. If you want to calm your mind and get into a zen-zone, do this breathing technique! That said, I would recommend this one on a day off or when you don't plan to go back to studying - only because you'll be so zen that you might not want to go back to work. It's especially good for managing performance anxiety or before you go to bed and it's bound to help you get a good night's sleep.

1. Place your your thumbs inside each ear.

2. Inhale.

3. As you exhale, hum the sound, "mmmmm".

4. Inhale.

5. Repeat the sound "mmmm".

Not too hard, right? Try it out.

Meditation:
A Powerful Tool To Improve
Your Cognition and Performance

We've all heard that meditation is amazing for focus, but did you ever wonder how it works on the brain to get those results? A study team through Harvard University found that eight weeks of Mindfulness-Based Stress Reduction (MBSR), which includes practicing mindfulness meditation, can change the structure of the brain by increasing cortical thickness in the hippocampus, the brain's center that governs learning and memory.

The researchers compared brain scans of 20 experienced meditators to those of 15 non-meditators. Brain scans revealed that the meditators boasted increased thickness in parts of the brain that deal with attention and processing sensory input. A pretty important revelation I'd say for taking an exam where processing of information is so important.

Evidence from meditation and the brain studies showed that certain areas of the brain play roles in emotion regulation and self-referential processing with decreases in brain cell volume in the amygdala, which is responsible for fear, anxiety, and stress, indicating that meditation not only changes the brain, but it changes our subjective perception and feelings as well.

In a randomized control trial where researchers from the University of Santa Barbara looked at two groups scheduled to take the Graduate Record Exam (GRE), one that did a two-week mindfulness training course and the other that enrolled in a nutrition course, both groups practiced daily. The mindfulness group had breathing and meditation practices and the nutrition group logged their daily food intake.

What do you think they found? You guessed it if you think they found that the mindfulness group had significantly improved cognitive performance on the GRE and working memory capacity, while reducing distracting thoughts over the nutrition group.

I hope this has convinced you that meditation can help you both with knowledge and memory, as well as processing and reducing stress and performance anxiety. It's the complete package - I hope you're sold to try it out and I'm here to support you in doing it.

Conclusion: Embracing Calm and Confidence through Yoga Therapy

Our professional and personal lives are often punctuated by moments that demand peak performance. It's easy for performance anxiety to seize control, leaving us in a state of unease. However, my experiences as a dietitian and a Yoga Therapist have illuminated the path to conquering this anxiety.

By infusing Yoga Therapy into the journey of my students preparing for dietetics board exams, I witnessed profound transformations. The practice of yoga, with its empowering asanas and calming pranayama techniques, became a powerful ally against test anxiety. These methods not only nurtured physical well-being but also instilled a newfound sense of calm and self-assuredness.

However, I couldn't ignore the striking parallel between their test anxiety and my own experience during my 500-hour yoga teacher training. It was a stark reminder that performance anxiety is a universal challenge, one that transcends professions and backgrounds. If I could offer one piece of wisdom, it would be this: don't underestimate the potency of meditation, pranayama, and yoga nidra (yogic sleep) in preparing for significant milestones. These practices are the keys to unlocking a reservoir of calm and confidence that can carry you to success.

As we navigate the chapters of our lives, let's remember the invaluable gift of Yoga Therapy in taming the anxiety that often accompanies performance. It is my hope that this chapter serves as a guiding light, illuminating a path toward a balanced, grounded, and confident approach to life's most critical moments.

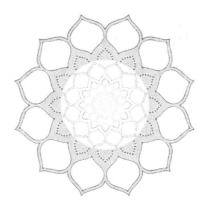

Imagine if everyone was going to a yoga therapist. Someone goes to a hospice, hospital, community center or a veteran's community. Have you got a C-IAYT?

~Leigh, C-IAYT

Harmony Unveiled: Nurturing the Flame Through Ayurvedic Nutrition

Ilene Cohen, MS, RDN, CLT, CDCES, C-IAYT

Embark on an immersive and enlightening journey into the rich tapestry of Ayurvedic well-being, where each pillar serves as a guiding light towards holistic harmony and vitality. Begin your journey with mindful movement, where the art of asana and poses becomes a gateway to physical strength, flexibility, and inner peace. Delve further into the realm of tranquility as pranayama and meditation unveil the profound serenity that lies within, offering respite from the ceaseless chatter of the mind and fostering a deep connection to the present moment. As the exploration continues, explore the cornerstone of Ayurvedic Nutrition, where the delicate balance of tastes and nourishment is meticulously curated to support optimal health and vitality. Explore the nuances of the six tastes, from the sweet embrace of nourishment to the refreshing zest of sourness, each offering a unique contribution to the symphony of flavors that nourish the body and soul. Unlock the therapeutic potential of herbs and spices, as their aromatic alchemy infuses each dish with healing properties and sensory delight. Discover the revered status of Ghee, the liquid gold of Ayurveda, revered for its nourishing qualities and versatile applications.

Throughout this immersive exploration, each section on tastes, spices, and recipes serves as a portal into a world where flavor and nourishment converge, inviting you to savor the abundance of holistic well-being. Nourish your body, mind, and spirit through the nurturing embrace of Ayurvedic care, harmonizing the intricate dance of your inner landscape and cultivating a radiant state of holistic health and vitality.

Ayurvedic Nutrition for Performance Anxiety

In my journey to alleviate performance anxiety through holistic practices, Ayurveda has emerged as a profound pillar in the pursuit of balance and well-being. Ayurveda, an ancient system of medicine originating from India, revolves around the concept of doshas – the three fundamental energies that govern our physical and mental characteristics. These doshas, known as Vata, Pitta, and Kapha, embody unique combinations of the five elements—earth, water, fire, air, and ether—and determine our individual constitution, or Prakruti.

As I enter into the holistic practices for alleviating performance anxiety, Ayurveda emerges as a profound pillar, intricately woven into the fabric of a balanced and harmonious life. Ayurveda, often referred to as the "science of life," is the sister science to yoga, seamlessly complementing its principles and extending its therapeutic reach. In the context of this Yoga Therapy book, Ayurveda becomes a guiding light, illuminating the path towards inner equilibrium and well-being.

At the heart of Ayurveda lies the understanding that our health is not merely the absence of disease, but a state of balance between our body, mind, and spirit. It recognizes the unique constitution of each individual, known as the dosha, and tailors its principles accordingly. Ayurveda views health as a dynamic interplay of the three doshas—Vata, Pitta, and Kapha—and their inherent qualities.

Vata, characterized by the elements of air and ether, governs movement and communication. Physically, Vata individuals tend to have a lighter frame, quick minds, and a propensity for dry skin. Emotionally, they may be creative and enthusiastic, but may also experience anxiety and restlessness. Mentally, Vata types are quick learners, but may struggle with focus.

Pitta, a passionate combination of fire and water, governs transformation and metabolism. Pitta individuals typically have a medium build, sharp intellect, and may be prone to sensitive skin. Emotionally, they exhibit passion and intensity, but imbalances may lead to irritability and perfectionism. Mentally, Pitta types are sharp, organized, and goal-oriented.

Kapha, grounded in earth and water elements, governs structure and stability. Physically, Kapha individuals tend to have a sturdy build, smooth skin, and a slower metabolism. Emotionally, they are calm and nurturing, but imbalances can lead to lethargy and attachment. Mentally, Kapha types are steady, compassionate, and methodical.

Understanding the unique qualities and tendencies of each dosha is crucial in the journey toward balance and well-being. It's about aligning our lifestyle, including nutrition, with our inherent nature to foster harmony within.

To bring the doshas into harmony, Ayurvedic nutrition plays a pivotal role. The key lies in understanding the six tastes and incorporating specific herbs and spices into our diet. Each taste—sweet, sour, salty, bitter, pungent, and astringent—plays a vital role in creating a balanced meal that caters to our unique constitution.

Let the tastes, spices, and meal timing become your allies in cultivating balance, confidence, and enhanced performance.

My Ayurvedic Odyssey

My voyage into the profound realm of Ayurveda has been nothing short of a transformative odyssey, threading the ancient wisdom of this holistic science into the tapestry of my wellness journey. It all began with my initiation into the world of yoga during my 200-hour yoga teacher training at YogaWorks in New York City. Little did I know that this would be the first stepping stone toward a deeper understanding of Ayurveda and its interconnectedness with yoga.

During my foundational training at YogaWorks, the seeds of curiosity were sown, and the roots of holistic well-being began to take hold. As I delved into the integrated science of Hatha, Tantra, and Ayurveda at ISHTA Yoga, a profound shift occurred. ISHTA became more than an acronym; it became a gateway to a profound understanding of how the principles of yoga, tantra, and Ayurveda harmoniously dance together to foster a balanced and vibrant existence.

ISHTA Yoga, with its emphasis on the integration of these ancient sciences, provided the fertile ground for my Ayurvedic studies to flourish. The teachings of Hatha yoga laid the foundation for mindful movement, Tantra illuminated the path of self-awareness and connection, and Ayurveda emerged as the guiding light for holistic health and balance.

As I delved deeper into the intricacies of Ayurveda, the science of life unfolded like a rich tapestry, revealing the intricate threads of doshas, tastes, and the art of mindful living. The philosophy of Ayurveda became more than a study—it became a way of life, guiding my choices on and off the mat. The wisdom embedded in Ayurveda transformed not only my personal well-being but also fueled my passion to share this holistic approach with others seeking harmony in their lives.

Through ISHTA Yoga's immersive Ayurvedic studies, I was able to bridge the ancient wisdom of Ayurveda with the contemporary practices of yoga, creating a synthesis that resonated with the essence of balance and holistic living. This journey has not only shaped my understanding of well-being, but has also become the guiding force in crafting "The Three Pillars of Serenity: Yoga for Performance Mastery," a program that encapsulates the synergies of Ayurvedic movement, stillness and calm, and mindful nutrition.

Venturing into the heart of Ayurveda, I discovered Pratima Spa in New York—a sanctuary where Ayurvedic sessions and massages became integral to my well-being. From Abhyanga to Shirodhara and Nasya, each treatment left a profound impact. Inspired, I embraced Ayurvedic skincare, witnessing the transformative effects on my skin with clay masks, cleansers, and essential oils.

In 2021, after the pandemic hiatus, I found Surya Spa in Santa Monica—a haven a few blocks away from my apartment. Martha, the spa's Ayurvedic practitioner and owner, guided me through a personalized journey, unraveling my vata-pitta dosha imbalances.

The combined Abhyanga and Shirodhara massage became my cherished ritual, complemented by delicious Ayurvedic lunches featuring dahl, fresh organic vegetables, and delectable Surya bread.

Immersing myself in a 7-day Panchakarma experience at Surya Spa proved a transformative part of my journey to self-discovery. The cleanse, followed by customized treatments, including Bhastis, left me rejuvenated and optimistic. Inspired to dig deeper, I enrolled in an Ayurvedic nutrition continuing education program for Registered Dietitians, unlocking a new realm of knowledge.

This transformative journey led me to explore Ayurvedic Health counselor programs. At SYTAR, the Symposium on Yoga Therapy and Research, Kerala Ayurveda Academy's curriculum stood out, capturing my attention. Now enrolled in their Ayurvedic Health counselor program, I eagerly anticipate integrating Ayurvedic tools into my role as a Yoga Therapist and Registered Dietitian nutritionist. This fusion of ancient wisdom and modern expertise is set to enrich the experiences of my students and clients, weaving Ayurveda into the fabric of both my businesses. As I tread this path, I am fueled by the excitement of sharing the profound benefits of Ayurveda with those who seek balance and holistic well-being.

This transformative expedition into Ayurveda has been a soul-nourishing experience, and I am eager to share the wisdom gleaned from this journey to empower others on their path to holistic wellness and performance mastery. The fusion of yoga and Ayurveda is not just a philosophy—it's a living, breathing practice that invites us to embrace the richness of our own existence and thrive in the dance of balance and well-being.

The Three Pillars of Serenity:
Yoga for Performance Mastery

Embarking on the transformative journey, enter "Serenity Flow: Yoga for Performance Mastery," my program that seamlessly integrates three pillars to cultivate a harmonious blend of physical vitality, mental resilience, and emotional balance. Each pillar stands as a cornerstone, offering a comprehensive approach to alleviating performance anxiety and embracing a life of serenity and confidence.

Pillar 1.

Ayurvedic Movement: Unleashing the Power of Asana and Poses

In the realm of Ayurvedic movement, the magic unfolds through the art of asana or yoga poses. Tailored to your unique dosha, these movements harmonize with your body's natural rhythm, promoting flexibility, strength, and balance. Whether you embody the grounding stillness of Kapha, the fiery precision of Pitta, or the creative flow of Vata, Ayurvedic movement becomes a personalized dance that awakens the body's potential and instills a sense of grounding and fluidity.

Pillar 2.

Stillness and Calm: Elevating the Mind through Pranayama and Meditation

---

Diving into the second pillar, we embrace the transformative power of stillness and calm. Through the practice of pranayama (breath control) and meditation, we journey inward to cultivate a tranquil mind. The rhythmic dance of the breath aligns with the Doshic clock, balancing Vata's restlessness, Pitta's intensity, and Kapha's calm. Meditation becomes the compass guiding us through the ebb and flow of thoughts, fostering mental clarity, emotional resilience, and a profound sense of peace.

Completing the triad of serenity, Ayurvedic nutrition serves as the foundation for nourishing the body and mind. Through the lens of the six tastes and the magic of Ayurvedic herbs and spices, we craft meals that not only tantalize the taste buds but also support optimal digestion, vibrant energy, and emotional balance. Whether it's the grounding sweetness of a date or the invigorating warmth of black pepper, each flavor becomes a note in the symphony of well-being, fostering a balanced and radiant self.

Together, these three pillars create a holistic haven for those seeking to conquer performance anxiety and embrace a life infused with serenity and confidence. "Serenity Flow: Yoga for Performance Mastery" beckons you to step onto the path of self-discovery, where Ayurvedic movement, stillness and calm, and mindful nutrition converge to unlock your true potential—a life of serenity, balance, and performance mastery.

The Symphony of Flavors: Ayurveda's Six Tastes Unveiled

In Ayurvedic nutrition, the concept of the six tastes plays a pivotal role in creating well-balanced and health-promoting meals. These tastes—sweet, sour, salty, bitter, pungent, and astringent—extend beyond merely flavor and are believed to have profound effects on our physical, mental, and emotional well-being. Let's consider each taste, understanding their qualities and the foods that embody them.

1.

Sweet Taste (Madhura):

The sweet taste nurtures the body and soothes the soul, offering comfort and satisfaction.

Qualities: Nourishing, grounding, and satisfying.

Foods: Fruits like bananas, mangoes, and dates; root vegetables like sweet potatoes; grains such as rice and wheat; and sweeteners like honey and maple syrup.

2.

Sour Taste (Amla):

The sour taste offers refreshing and stimulating qualities while promoting digestion.

Qualities: Refreshing, stimulating, and promotes digestion.

Foods: Citrus fruits like lemons and oranges; sour berries; fermented foods like yogurt and pickles; and vinegar.

3.

Salty Taste (Lavana):

The salty taste provides hydrating effects, warming properties, and enhances the overall flavor.

Qualities: Hydrating, warming, and enhances flavor.

Foods: Sea salt; salty vegetables like celery and seaweed; salty cheeses; and naturally salty foods like miso and tamari.

4.
Bitter Taste (Tikta):

Embrace the bitter taste known for its detoxifying and cooling qualities, serving as a digestive aid.

Qualities: Detoxifying, cooling, and aids digestion.

Foods: Leafy greens like kale and spinach; bitter gourds; herbs like neem and turmeric; and dark chocolate.

5.
Pungent Taste (Katu):

Experience the warming and stimulating qualities of the pungent taste (Katu), which also enhances metabolism.

Qualities: Warming, stimulating, and energizing.

Foods: Spices like black pepper, ginger, and garlic; radishes; onions; and certain cruciferous vegetables.

6.
Astringent Taste (Kashaya):

The astringent taste offers stability and soothing benefits, especially in times of heightened stress.

Qualities: Drying, cooling, and tones tissues.

Foods: Legumes like lentils and beans; fruits like apples and pomegranates; vegetables like cauliflower and broccoli; and certain grains like quinoa.

Understanding the balance of these tastes in your meals is akin to orchestrating a symphony for your well-being. The sweet taste provides comfort, the sour and salty tastes stimulate digestion, the bitter taste aids detoxification, the pungent taste enhances metabolism, and the astringent taste tones tissues. A harmonious blend of these tastes not only tantalizes the taste buds, but also fosters balance in the body and mind, promoting optimal health and vitality.

Aromatic Alchemy:
Discovering Ayurvedic Herbs and Spices

As we delve deeper into the world of Ayurvedic nutrition, we encounter herbs and spices like hing, saffron, turmeric, cardamom, and cinnamon, each with its unique set of attributes. These spices, when used mindfully, contribute to balancing the doshas and promoting overall well-being.

One spice that stands out in Ayurvedic nutrition, particularly in its impact on blood sugar levels and its connection to performance anxiety, is cinnamon. Beyond its aromatic and flavorful essence, cinnamon has the remarkable ability to balance blood sugar levels. This is essential for maintaining a stable energy supply to the brain and body, ultimately influencing our mood and cognitive function. The steadying effect on blood sugar levels can be a game-changer in the realm of performance anxiety, helping to curb the rollercoaster of emotions and thoughts that often accompany stressful situations.

Furthermore, it possesses energizing properties, offering the right dose of alertness and mental stamina to enhance overall performance and build confidence. It's like a harmonious dance of tastes and spices that not only pleases the palate, but also supports a balanced and energized state of being.

In the realm of fertility, bay leaf emerges as a powerful ally. Known for its positive effects on motility, it can be a valuable addition to your culinary arsenal. Furthermore, spices play a crucial role in digestion, with black pepper taking the spotlight. Its warming and pungent taste stimulate the appetite, enhancing

Agni, or digestive fire, which is essential for overall well-being.

⇒ *The effect of cinnamon supplementation on glycemic control in patients with type 2 diabetes or with polycystic ovary syndrome: an umbrella meta-analysis on interventional meta-analyses.Diabetol Metab Syndr 15, 127 (2023). https://doi.org/10.1186/s13098-023-01057-2*

Understanding the needs of specific doshas, mustard seeds, with their heating and pungent properties, become a valuable resource. Particularly beneficial for Kapha and Vata imbalances, they contribute to heart health and skin well-being. Additionally, mustard seeds exhibit analgesic properties, providing relief from pain, gas, bloating, and nausea.

Coriander seeds, a staple in Ayurvedic nutrition, cleanse the urinary system and prove beneficial for conditions like UTIs. A tea made from coriander seeds can be a soothing remedy for painful urination and excessive thirst.

In the pursuit of balance for Vata and Kapha, cumin takes center stage. Rich in phytoestrogens, it supports the reproductive system. It's worth noting that while adjwan might be unsuitable for those with epilepsy, cumin serves as a viable alternative for addressing this condition.

Ginger, whether dried or fresh, emerges as a versatile spice with numerous benefits. Its warming properties make it an excellent bioavailability enhancer and a supportive aid for the reproductive system. A simple concoction of sliced ginger, lemon juice, and Himalayan pink salt before meals can kindle your digestive fire.

Garlic, though potent, requires careful consideration. Its heating nature makes it suitable for Vata-Kapha imbalances, while caution is advised for Pitta. In medicinal applications, garlic can be beneficial for congestion, cough, and reducing cholesterol. Its lactation-enhancing properties make it a valuable resource for blocked breastfeeding ducts.

Fennel, with its mild sweet taste, proves soothing for Pitta and beneficial for the female reproductive system. It's a versatile herb that finds a place in Indian restaurants as sweetened candied fennel, offering relief for menstrual cramps.

Fenugreek, renowned for its legendary aphrodisiac properties, also acts as a galactagogue, and has been claimed to enhance breast milk production. Its bitter taste makes it suitable for addressing anorexia, while its ability to defend against diabetes underscores its multifaceted benefits.

Culinary Harmony:
Ayurvedic Meal Planning for Holistic Wellness

Now, let's explore some Ayurvedic meal plan ideas designed to embrace the six tastes and harness the benefits of herbs and spices. For breakfast, imagine a nourishing bowl of oat or rice cereal infused with a blend of soaked, cooked almonds for grounding, cooked dates for sweetness, and vibrant blueberries for a touch of tartness. This combination not only kick starts your day with a mix of tastes, but also provides sustained energy.

As lunch takes center stage as the most substantial meal, consider a balanced plate with a variety of tastes. Picture a meal with a base of whole grains like quinoa or brown rice, accompanied by a colorful array of vegetables, both cooked and raw, to ensure a mix of flavors and textures. Add a protein source like lentils or tofu for substance and a dash of spices like cumin, coriander, and turmeric for both taste and Ayurvedic benefits.

As the day winds down, let dinner be a lighter affair. Opt for a simple and easily digestible soup or stew, incorporating seasonal vegetables, lentils, and a gentle blend of herbs and spices like ginger and fennel. This allows the body to prepare for restful sleep without the burden of heavy digestion.

Speaking of sleep, Ayurveda places great importance on the doshic clock, recognizing that each dosha predominates during specific times of the day. Evening, governed by Kapha, is ideal for winding down and preparing for a restful night. Thus, aligning your meals with the doshic clock can promote optimal digestion and overall well-being.

Ghee:
Liquid Gold in Ayurveda

In Ayurveda, ghee, or clarified butter, is often hailed as "liquid gold" due to its magical and tremendous healing potential. To make ghee, butter is gently simmered to remove impurities, leaving behind a rich, golden substance. This process enhances its digestibility and allows it to carry the healing properties of herbs and spices deep into the tissues. Ghee is prized for its ability to lubricate the digestive tract, support nutrient absorption, and kindle the digestive fire (Agni). Its unique composition makes it suitable for all three doshas—Vata, Pitta, and Kapha. For those following a vegan diet, coconut oil can be a wonderful substitute in Ayurvedic recipes, offering a similar nourishing quality with a delightful coconut flavor. Ghee plays a crucial role in Ayurvedic cooking, contributing to both the taste and therapeutic benefits of the meals we enjoy.

Ayurvedic Breakfast Bowl:
Oat or Rice Cereal with Almonds, Dates, and Blueberries

Ingredients:

- 1 cup rolled oats or cooked rice
- 1 teaspoon ghee (clarified butter)
- 1/4 cup almonds, soaked and cooked
- 3-4 dates, pitted and chopped
- 1/2 cup fresh blueberries
- 1/2 teaspoon cinnamon powder
- A pinch of salt
- Optional: honey or maple syrup for sweetness

Instructions:

1. Cook the oats or rice according to package instructions.

2. In a pan, warm the ghee over low heat. Add the soaked and cooked almonds, tossing them until they become slightly golden.

3. Mix the cooked almonds, chopped dates, blueberries, cinnamon powder, and a pinch of salt into the oats or rice.

4. Drizzle with honey or maple syrup for added sweetness, if desired.

5. Stir well and enjoy a grounding and energizing breakfast.

Ayurvedic Lunch Plate:
Quinoa or Brown Rice with Vegetables and Lentils

Ingredients:

- 1 tablespoon ghee
- 1 teaspoon cumin powder
- 1 teaspoon coriander powder
- 1/2 teaspoon turmeric powder
- 1 cup quinoa or brown rice, cooked
- Mixed vegetables (carrots, broccoli, bell peppers, zucchini, etc.)
- 1/2 cup cooked lentils or tofu cubes
- Salt to taste
- Fresh cilantro for garnish

Instructions:

1. In a pan, heat ghee over medium heat. Add cumin, coriander, and turmeric powder, allowing them to release their aromas.

2. Add the mixed vegetables and sauté until they are tender yet retain their crunch.

3. Stir in the cooked lentils or tofu cubes, ensuring they are coated with the spices.

4. Serve this vegetable and lentil mix over a bed of quinoa or brown rice.

5. Garnish with fresh cilantro and enjoy a flavorful, balanced lunch.

Ayurvedic Dinner:
Healing Kitchari

Ingredients:

- 1/2 cup basmati rice
- 1/2 cup yellow split mung beans (split yellow lentils)
- 1 tablespoon ghee or coconut oil
- 1 teaspoon cumin seeds
- 1 teaspoon mustard seeds
- 1/2 teaspoon fennel seeds
- 1/2 teaspoon grated ginger
- 1/2 cup mixed vegetables (carrots, peas, zucchini)
- 1/2 teaspoon turmeric powder
- 1/2 teaspoon ground coriander
- 4 cups water or vegetable broth
- Salt to taste
- Fresh cilantro for garnish
- Optional: squeeze of fresh lemon juice

Instructions:

* Rinse the basmati rice and yellow split mung beans thoroughly.

* In a pot, heat ghee or coconut oil over medium heat. Add cumin seeds, mustard seeds, fennel seeds, and grated ginger. Allow them to sizzle and release their aroma.

* Add the mixed vegetables, turmeric powder, ground coriander, and a pinch of salt. Sauté for a few minutes until the vegetables begin to soften.

* Stir in the rinsed rice and mung beans, coating them in the spice mixture.

* Pour in the water or vegetable broth, bring to a boil, then reduce heat to simmer. Cover and cook until the rice and beans are tender, and the consistency is creamy.

* Adjust salt to taste and garnish with fresh cilantro. Squeeze a bit of fresh lemon juice if desired.

* Serve warm and savor the nourishing and balancing qualities of Ayurvedic kitchari.

In Ayurveda, balance isn't just about what you eat, but also how you live. Embracing the wisdom of the doshic clock, prioritizing a substantial lunch, and keeping dinner light can contribute to a harmonious lifestyle. So, as you embark on this Ayurvedic journey, let the tastes, spices, and meal timing become your allies in cultivating balance, confidence, and enhanced performance in both mind and body.

I can't wait for you to embark on this journey with me. The Ayurvedic dosha assessment isn't just about labels; it's about uncovering your unique blueprint for well-being. So, are you ready to discover your dosha and receive personalized tips to enhance your daily life? Let's dive in together and embrace the wisdom of Ayurveda, tailoring our approach to Yoga Therapy and nutrition to the beautiful symphony of our own unique constitution. An Ayurvedic dosha assessment can unlock a world of insights that will empower your journey towards balance and radiant well-being.

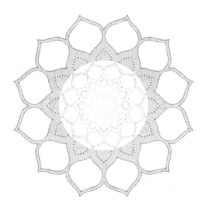

Yoga Therapy requires not only that you start as a yoga teacher, but then you continue on and do an additional 800 hours of training. That 800 hours includes clinical hours. It's always spread over two years to make sure that it's not this rushed thing. Only a percentage of those hours can be online. There also needs to be that in-person component. It has a pretty high level of rigor.

~ Ann, C-IAYT

Integrating Soul-in-Medicine with Your Yoga Therapy Path

Annie Kay, MS, RDN, E-RYT500, C-IAYT

As you navigate your transformative journey of yoga, Annie shares how an examined life can help you navigate life's difficult personal and professional situations. Through her experiences and insights, she reminds you to seek sanctuary in the solitude of sādhanā, the sacred daily practice of yoga. The chapter navigates the intricate balance between love, duty, and creative expression, drawing parallels to the Hindu goddess Sarasvatī and her creative nature, at times in conflict with the needs of family and friends.

You can embrace the guiding questions your best teachers provide. Those questions are keys that can help unlock your inner temple and allow for a deeper understanding of yourself and your Yoga Therapy. Annie shares her intricate dance between love and yoga, understanding their entangled essence of soul-in-medicine. Explore her challenges and the lessons she encountered in the world of yoga teaching, from personal entanglements to ethical considerations.

You can witness the healing power of yoga in the lives of individuals as they are guided through chronic metabolic medical conditions. Join this journey into the integration of yoga, spirituality, and Western medicine. Your Yoga Therapy path can be one of self-discovery and sacred healing as you serve others and have a good time. Finally, Annie provides an invitation to connect, and a few questions for self-inquiry.

Namaste.

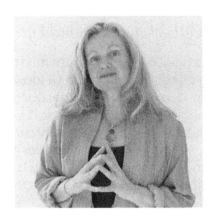

Annie B. Kay MS, RDN, E-RYT500, C-IAYT, inspires health professionals seeking soul-in-medicine, and women in the second half of life seeking holistic solutions to chronic metabolic issues. Her method celebrates your unique life journey, unearths what fuels your life force, and then empowers you to build a more balanced, happier, and integrated life.

Annie is a Registered Licensed Dietitian Nutritionist, Certified Yoga Therapist, and shamanic herbalist who writes, speaks, and has a private practice in Massachusetts. She holds a BS in Nutritional Biochemistry from Cornell, an MS in Nutrition Communications from Boston University, and numerous certifications in integrative health.

Formerly Lead Nutritionist at Kripalu, the largest holistic education center in the US, Annie now speaks and leads programs online and internationally. Her books include *Every Bite Is Divine*, and *Yoga & Diabetes* published with the American Diabetes Association, plus a CE program on Yoga Therapy and metabolism for health professionals.

www.anniebkay.com

Gifts of an Examined Life

In the dark early morning, a family of deer munch on the remains of summer's flowers as seen through the window of my quiet living room. I roll out my mat as I've done for decades and turn my attention to my physical body – this body, soft yet strong, filled with nicks and scars, this one I live my life through. Questions arise to frame the inquiry. What new ache or familiar tension, what sadness or joy, are in here today? How will my body's messages guide or inform my day and suggest my medicine now?

Finding Sanctuary in Sādhanā

Practice (Sādhanā), the solitary routine of yoga, is a sanctuary. It's a sacred place I inhabit that allows me to explore the hidden landscapes inside my body and soul. My solace lay not in the world outside but in the stillness within. I find peace in the soft golden pink of the dawn - when the world is yet to awaken to its bustle. In the tranquility of that hour, I flow deep into the rhythm of my breath, hear the whispers of my own heart, and sense a unity in the universe, and the essence of yoga. It is a prayer with a quest for self-realization, a slow and continual process of shedding layers and rediscovering my inner light. As the day brightens it embraces me. I have today's compass in hand.

Sādhanā is a central practice of my examined life.

This Integrating Path

This winding journey, on the path of darning and darning again what has been rendered – torn by us – is as long as life, it seems. And yet. I've witnessed wholeness and hope you have too. In the shine of another's eye. In your own tears – of joy, of woe and connection.

I'm a Sarasvatī (the Hindu goddess of creativity and study) woman. The creative daughter of a wise and powerful father, I'd rather be writing, reading in solitude, or teaching a small group than hobnobbing at a party any day. The goddess Sarasvatī dresses in white, sits on a lotus, and travels on a large white swan, a symbol of transcendence.

Her four arms hold a Pustaka (book of scriptures, representing universal wisdom of the Vedas), a mala (meditation beads representing inner reflection), a water pot (representing the purifying power of separating right from wrong, and the water represents soma, the drink of liberating knowledge), and a musical instrument called a vīṇā (symbolizing creative expression and sacred rhythm).

There is a story of Sarasvatī that resonates with my own. Her proud and loving husband expected her beautiful presence at a banquet, but as the festivities commenced, she was nowhere to be found. Where was she? Upstairs in the library, of course, lost in her latest book and note-taking. He was annoyed and accused her of not caring for him or their guests, though of course she did. Her nature, however, drew her to learn and ponder ideas in solitude. She lost track of time in the stories and ideas. How might he draw her back? Rhythm. Just play a bit of music, and she can't resist the call to move.

The pull between loving and caring for my family and the draw of creative expression has been a central professional theme with uncanny timing. In the end, I've chosen love, imperfectly, every time, all the while feeling the pull of that upstairs library or classroom and the creative expression it holds. My Yoga Therapy path, my sādhanā, helps me ease the tensions between seeming competing forces in my life.

For example, after five years of writing, my first book, *Every Bite Is Divine* was published and it was time to promote it. That same winter my beloved father fell ill. He passed away that spring after a short vicious struggle with cancer. In grief, I canceled the planned book tour. That took the air out of the endeavor like a deflating balloon. Years later I launched my first independent international retreat in Costa Rica, and just before I left my husband contracted an especially nasty cancer. I traveled and taught numb with grief, grateful to his sister who took my vigil those weeks. It's a gray joy.

A choice, with tension – love or the energetic satisfaction and demands of public creative expression. Yoga helps me dance between them.

Guiding Questions: Unlocking Inner Landscapes

I've always found yoga more profound than physical exercise. The perfect headstand lost its appeal for me early in my yoga journey. My teachers gave me the gift of finding a deeper connection within myself, a connection that transcends my ordinary relative world and ventures into the velvety realm of the absolute, the realm of the soul.

We all yearn for quick solutions and tidy lessons.

However, learning to live the questions without ruminating too much on the answers, has served me well. Patience, grasshopper. Answers come along with living and choosing to live. They come.

The gentle inclusive language of my teachers - Barbara Benagh and Patricia Walden in Boston, Bhavani Maki in Kauai, Pam Montgomery in Vermont, and my mentors at Kripalu - was a guiding light on my path inward. Yet, their true teaching skill – what impacted the trajectory of my life off the mat - wasn't so much the postures, sequences, or even the philosophical teachings themselves. It was their presence and the questions they asked.

They each understood that the right question could unlock profound inner chambers. So it was with me.

Through so many hours of practice, Swami Kripalu smiling down from an altar or wall over us, my Kripalu mentors Aruni or Kavi would ask, "What are you holding that no longer serves you? Can you let a bit of it go with each exhale?" Then deeper and more contemplative, "What would your body, your heart or belly, say if it could speak freely? If you could listen deeply and fully hear it?" These teachers, with these and other questions, taught me how to live an examined life.

These questions taught me how to turn down the static of external pressures, listen to my heart, and choose my way. Moment by moment, day by day.

As my teachership developed, I also planted questions in the soil of those I served. "Can you feel the pulse of energy – of life, of prāṇa (vitality) - in your body? What is the quality of your energy at this moment?", I ask. "Based on that energy, what will nourish and rebalance you now?"

Navigating Your Inner Temple

Wise woman Sally Kempton took me deep into the velvet cave of my own heart. She taught me how to tolerate grief and discomforts, to learn to linger there, and to get to know my inner landscape.

The quiet terrain of your thoughts, emotions, and spirit is a spark of the divine. In yoga, we often say that our bodies are temples, but it is in the silent inner temple that the gems of yoga reside. In the quietude of meditative practice, you just may find a depth of peace that cannot be found in the external spinning world. The true journey of yoga is one of solitude, but it's a voyage inward that can help you live fully, regardless of who, what, or where you are.

If you feel the sacredness of sādhanā – and you teach others – sharing your experience can be an invitation to them to do the same.

I've found teaching spirit is mostly about creating a safe space for its inclusion. Tell your students how you create space for it, how you hold it, and tend it or not. Learn to hold silent witness in those you serve.

At Kripalu, we held share circles for the sacred relational experience of witness and presence. A collection of souls gathered, and after a body-based centering, I asked, "What's going on for you?" After a few sober breaths, I deepen the invitation with "What is really going on for you?"

We witness reports from the inner temples of those in the circle without interrupting or dialogue. We practice presence by bringing ourselves fully to the circle and speaking the truth as best we can. There are tears and profound silence. Each soul shares from within, their joy and woe. Sacredness arises from these gatherings nearly every time. I continue the honor of holding souls, planting seeds, witnessing, and being present, almost every single day.

Love, Yoga, and Developing Helpful Boundaries

Tangled like an inner inheritance, I've always had faith that love and yoga are both so large that I can travel with them all my life, on an endless soul-filled breath. So it has been, with long kumbhak (breath suspension) between.

Like many initiates, I fell in love with both the practice of yoga and my first yoga teacher. It was a whirl of energy at the time. With perspective, I've learned that it was a distorted romantic love that got entangled with my appreciation for the activation of emotional and spiritual growth. I was living in Central Square (a hippie haven dubbed the Center of the Universe) in Cambridge, MA. I worked as the Osteoporosis Awareness Program Director for the Massachusetts Department of Public Health (DPH) in Boston.

A goofy sweet guy with a beautiful body was at the center of my yoga initiation. He was gentle and kind with a habit of bedding his students. He activated me into yoga, a practice that has guided every dimension of my life. Yoga activation is a heady but tender time. That expansion can be taken advantage of – perhaps unwittingly – by teachers. Energetic expansion and romantic love easily become entangled and confused. The student inevitably loses something, and when my first yoga love didn't work out, I lost my practice and community in addition to my boyfriend. It's a complicated yet too common lesson in this perfectly imperfect world of yoga.

There are established ethics of working in the caring professions. Learning them early can save you time, and heartache. One ethical tenet is to resist the temptation of romantic relationships with your students or underlings.

After watching it unfold in myself and others, the careful guide rails that some organizations use for these tender situations can be helpful. If they're honored.

Iyengar yoginī (female practitioner) Patricia Walden, whose yogic alignment was a class unto itself, suggested I visit Kripalu. She saw that I yearned for a heart-centered soul-filled internal dance in my practice. My first yoga experience at Kripalu was Moon Series led by a strong gorgeous yoginī. She lengthened us slowly slowly forward, her voice a hand pressed lovingly into our low backs to guide our spines longer as we bowed, bending a forward knee to kiss our foreheads. Jānu śīrṣāsana (seated forward fold) asks us to bow to our practice. Of course, I fell madly for her, and sacred yoga in the cathedral of Kripalu's main hall. This time, my passion was channeled inward to fuel my sādhanā. Much better.

I put off becoming a yoga teacher for five years beyond feeling called to do so. I wanted to follow along the sacred transformative path of yoga and let it happen for a while – before turning it into a job. I grew up Catholic believing there was something more in sacred life though I wasn't sure just how it included me. Yoga gave me that big yes of inclusion with my first transformative moment. After 10 years of practice, I felt namaste (divinity within recognizing divinity in another) – perfectly imperfect yet undeniable. Regardless of my messy hair, jelly belly, or dumb-struck tendency when challenged, a fire ignited that burns bright in me to this day.

The Yoga-Clinical Interface

I fell in love with the voice, writing, and teaching of master languager Barbara Benagh, who could navigate her way behind your right kidney to relax a tiny muscle behind it. I began to study yoga seriously. Kripalu, Ashtanga, Iyengar-Hatha, and later Shamanic herbalism and alchemical plant medicine drew me like a moth to a flame. I've been weaving my passions of therapeutic nutritional biochemistry and Yoga Therapy together ever since.

Yoga is a long-term project in learning about relationships (in life and with your ever-evolving self).

My best teachers now are my clients and the lives they choose. Their dreams and effort inspire me. Their rambles along their rocky paths are what life is made of.

Plants are also generous teachers, especially the great White Pines on the land I tend. Working with plants completed an education I began as a nutritional biochemist at Cornell. Plants have taught me most of what I know about energy and nature. They take me deep into spirals of life, growth, death, and resprouting. They teach the alchemical spiral of transformation.

The tsunami of suffering that is relationship with food in America today, responds well to the mercy and integrating peace of Yoga Therapy.

I began to experiment, applying the philosophical tenets of yoga to myself and others, and found that my clients respond with relief and often, change. That realization launched my first book – *Every Bite Is Divine* – and much of my work since.

Teaching at the cusp of integration can be tricky. It requires being clear on the ever-shifting boundaries between Western clinical science, Eastern wisdom, and metaphysics.

We make students and clients aware of where we are, point by point, line by line as we navigate and re-discover these new-to-the-West soul-in-medicine lands. We find ways to be bold yet humble – to learn to say "I don't know" not as a defeat but as an invitation. We re-integrate what's been torn.

Metabolic health – how all the biochemistry in your body creates and uses energy – is an issue of our time. The diseases of metabolic health – heart disease, diabetes, thyroid diseases, and some cancers – reflect choices and so reflect who you are.

Healing metabolic disease requires self-examination. If you simply follow someone else's recipe, without compassionate self-reflection and customization, your chances I'm afraid, are only fair to middling.

Healing metabolic disease requires real-life change. That's hard to do.

In 2006 (nearly 20 years ago) I wrote a book-length CE program for dietitians and other nutrition pros called Yoga & Meditation: Tools for Weight Management. It's gone through three editions and I'm revamping it yet again as *Yoga, Meditation & Ayurveda: Therapeutic Tools for Metabolic Health* (Great Valley Publishing). *Every Bite is Divine: the balanced approach to enjoying eating, feeling healthy and happy, and getting to your natural weight*, is the trade version of the teachings. It's humbling to meet people who've gotten to know me through my writing. These tombs are scouts that reach a bit further out along my teaching path. Hopefully, they're a helping hand to others along theirs.

Work and Life Partners are Essential, and Students are Teachers

Kripalu was my full-time work home for seven wild and wonderful years. There were times I was on fire teaching amongst an amazing collection of colleagues channeling the divine together. Life at Kripalu was a kundalini path. The kundalini path contains a hearty dose of fire. Every few years there was a bonfire and the organization was reorganized. My mentors there said this hot churn had swirled for 35 years.

Kripalu gave me a platform and time to develop my passion for the healing gift of yoga into a stronger voice and a song. For that, I will ever be grateful. The fire of transformation singed me numerous times as we tumbled through those years. I cried, laid on the floor of my office, dusted myself off, laughed with colleagues, and danced again.

To see souls – by the thousands - drag themselves up from New York, or in from Boston, gray and exhausted on Sunday night, broke my heart wide open. Then over five days (I mostly taught mid-week programs), Kripalu did the magic that it does – I saw them shine up and pink up, their faces glowing by noontime Friday. It was thanks to chew chew chewing lots of kale, laughing, and moving through the devotional yoga of compassion, with lights out at ten. The morning call back to the mat came just before the misty mountain dawn.

My teacher-colleagues at Kripalu – Tarika, Martha, Aruni, Kavi, Lisa, Kathie and so many more – helped me form and reform the questions and build a capacity to cook in postures and life. Kripalu yoga explores our whole yogic being - with mercy and compassion - as a context for life's unfolding.

The discomfort of holding Vīrabhadrāsana 2 (Warrior 2), for example, arms extended, shoulders relaxed yet anything but quiet, exploring how to make this posture more about balance and resting on earthly lines of energy than about powering through and shakily grasping, is how life can feel. That shaky discomfort, a container for considering just how like life holding the pose (of beloved family and friends experiencing joys and tragedies) can be, is instructive. It taught me how to hold big emotions, and how discomfort naturally shifts and eases over time.

Our bodies can be superb integrators of experience should we choose to take that path. In my time at Kripalu and these years since, being with the questions my teachers gave me, and cooking in sādhanā, has helped me to develop faith in the unfolding of my own life. Everything that happens, guides my sacred path, growth, and highest aims.

Kripalu is filled with talented people doing gorgeous work, often under difficult circumstances. Spirit and commerce, done with integrity have been challenged, bent, and misconstrued in ways that can make it hard to trust. Navigating the fantasy world of retreat vacation while seeking can be so much fun, deeply touching, and downright hysterically funny. It can also burn your candle down, fast, to the quick. Compassion and mercy can be hard to find at the moments you need them most. As my Kripalu fire wained, heading back into my internal temple helped me move forward in my life.

One early morning during that time, as the sun rose in the Eastern sky, it lit me that familiar pink. The rose of Utthita Trikonasana (extended Triangle Pose) spiraled from my center point. I realized that life spirals too – in, as William Blake suggests – joy and woe, woven fine—clothing for the soul divine.

Trikonasana embodies dynamic balance. We root to reach, spiral, waver, and fall our way to strength and fullness. As I stretch and surrender, teetering on my furthest edge of comfort, I evolve. I feel where my aging body is weakening, and where my heart has made space for breath. I teach my song more fully now – and teach the integration of science and spirit in the ways I'd always imagined. Root and reach, sorrow and joy.

...But Give Your Adoration with Care

You may find that while our media-driven world loves a celebrity, many yearn for a refuge from the cacophony of performative voices. Your ability to perform can come in handy but never lose sight of the best interests of those you serve. It's about them. Remember your ethics of caring. The more worldly success you have, the more difficult it seems to avoid this particular corruption. There is sociopathic behavior on this trail. Activating students into yoga can feel fantastic for all involved and can be the basis for either big steps forward in understanding or more destructive cult-like behavior.

An awareness of who a teacher's work ultimately serves is important. The health and well-being of students or followers must be enhanced, and never compromised. If a teaching or practice does not honor the basics of well-being it is not helpful for anyone involved.

Mindful eating, for example, is a profoundly powerful practice that has transformed the way I and many nutritionists work with people who want to eat better but struggle. The practice helps you regulate your appetite to a great extent, and to deeply savor the miracle of bringing the energy of the sun and earth into your internal universe.

Meditative mindful eating can, if not taught properly, lead to chronic undereating and malnutrition. I've seen too many yoga teachers develop eating disorders because that powerful practice was taught as - just eat a whole lot less - rather than with health in mind, grounded in nutritional adequacy.

Unnecessary suffering due to uninformed or misguided teaching is, unfortunately, rampant. Choose your teachers with care.

Yoga Therapy as Soul-In-Medicine

It's a thrill to translate the gifts of yoga to those who suffer from chronic medical conditions; people who carry the scars and challenges of life in their bodies.

I lived on Nantucket for several years. My husband had a friend whom many on the island loved – carpenter and ever-chuckling creative genius Dell Wynn. Dell helped build our beautiful home, and came up with the hilarious business idea of 'rent a buddy'. He received a diagnosis of progressive Lou Gehrig's disease (ALS) in his prime. Dell had a strong yoga practice and was fit in his 50s. As he faded, he asked me to work with him. I remember holding my hand at his crown, talking him into one of his favorite postures, śīrṣāsana (headstand), as he sat immobile in his wheelchair. I could feel his energy body organizing around his Suṣumṇa nāḍī (central energetic channel), lengthening, and strengthening, as his mind took his withered body into the posture. We cried and admired the familiar sacred glow of yoga. It was a beautiful headstand.

Lifestyle medicine – eating a little better, moving a little more, practicing self-compassion, and learning to let go and lighten up about life – is the most powerful medicine we have today. I see people heal – from pre-diabetes, from serious gut imbalance, from pain and fatigue – every day, step by step, spiraling up (then down then up again) - with soul-in-medicine.

This Soul-in-Medicine Song I Sing

I love dietitians – smart, well-meaning, science-driven. Mind-body dietitians bring a range of integrative training and perspectives – family systems, qui gong, mindfulness, and more –to their integrative practice. Clinicians on this edge are threatened by being labeled "too woo woo" if they venture too far along the path of integration, while also being stand-ins for all that's wrong with medicine to more spirit-centric healers. It's yet another job for your inner temple.

In addition to my metabolic private practice, I've been happily offering webinars with a clinician publisher, Great Valley Publishing. Dietitians have told me my webinars give them goosebumps – tears! – to know that this sort of soul-in-medicine practice exists. Western science is evolving rapidly on the benefits and details of Yoga Therapy, including meditation and yogic breathing. The 'dose' of yoga and its effects is becoming apparent. Not surprisingly, more yoga and more support lead to better outcomes.

My passion is the complexities of metabolic health and how yoga can help with the chronic conditions of imbalanced metabolism. From thyroid issues, high blood pressure, and pre-diabetes to heart diseases, these issues are the sad fallout for the vast majority of Americans living our over-commercialized lives.

My vocation is to teach and mentor dietitians and other health professionals how to integrate sacred yoga into clinical protocols. We can weave food and plant-based soul into medically indicated lifestyles.

> Coaxing those for whom movement is a painful experience to reawaken flow through adaptive yoga practice can revolutionize medicine.

Yoga Therapist-clinicians can offer skillful movement, breath, and yoga philosophy as an adjunct medicine for every condition known to us.

Now, Your Path

> As you create your Western path for soul-in-medicine, remember the inclusion of the sacred in your integration. Bring it back, gently fight for it, it is critical. Regardless of what some call you, you're not "too woo-woo". You are a perfectly imperfect integrative practitioner.

Gather ye guides, traveler. Find those who help you ask the right questions to unlock your inner temple as you serve others. Those who know, teach and live by the ethics of caring even when it is inconvenient or unprofitable.

Advocate for the future inclusive of the sacred. Advocate for sacred yoga.

If this resonates with you, you can gather with me and a collection of souls seeking and creating soul-in-medicine. There's a seat for you around this fire.

Blessings for your journey.
Annie

Annie's Questions for Self-Inquiry

- What is your sādhanā? What takes you into your own inner temple?

- When you feel confused or overwhelmed, what can or do you do? What do you draw from or lean on?

- Do you know what your life mission is? If not, what brings you joy, and what are you most passionate about?

- Do you have a community of like-minded people? What might your ideal community be and feel like?

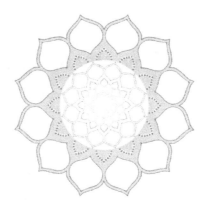

In the United States, one of the things that I'm really passionate and excited about is this idea that pain, whether it's mental, emotional or physical, is multifaceted. It has multiple causes. What you eat, if you exercise, if you don't, how much sleep you're getting, what kind of stress you're under. I'm excited that Yoga Therapy has the answers to that. We use a multifaceted intervention strategy.

~Amy, C-IAYT

A Military Yogi

Adhana McCarthy, MPAS, PA-C, C-IAYT

Follow the throughline of one woman's yoga journey from a community organizer at a Californian organic food co-op to soldier at an isolated base in the Iraqi war. Wanting to learn more about the Iraqi war, Adhana, joined the Army searching for an authentic experience. This complete U-turn on her life path, showed her not only how her worlds would collide, but how they would complement each other. As she filled the need for soldiers to practice yoga while deployed to the middle east, she discovered how yoga could help in the midst of grief, sadness and chaos.

Adhana pursued a career as a physician assistant and yoga therapist, weaving yoga into her medical practice. As she treated soldiers with stress, insomnia and pain, she realized that yoga was something to return to over and over again to develop resilience and mental toughness over her 20 year military career.

In this chapter, Adhana highlights the highs and lows of being a military yogi. She discusses the benefits of establishing a yoga practice in community and how creating a structure around health behaviors can make it easier for groups to make better health choices. Understanding that yoga is not a panacea, she does not neglect the challenges of maintaining a yoga practice in isolation. Ultimately, she highlights how yoga combined with positive relationships helped her to sustain a lasting personal transformation.

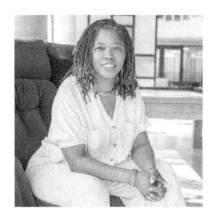

Adhana McCarthy, MPAS, PA-C, C-IAYT is an Army physician assistant, public health scholar, certified Yoga Therapist and certified life coach who has served in the military for 20 years. She works with leaders and high-risk professionals to help them regulate their nervous systems, so they can have clarity and courage during high-stakes situations and decrease the risk for burnout. She uses the tools of yoga, mindfulness and cognitive reframing to build personalized strategies to ease the anxious mind, quiet self-criticism, and improve personal leadership as they reach for big goals. She has taught internationally and works with military, medical professionals, and entrepreneurs.

Indeed, for a warrior, there is no better engagement than fighting for upholding of righteousness.

– Bhagavad Gita 2.31

Imagine a day where yoga training, and other health promoting behaviors are used to help cope with the stresses of military service. Imagine warfighters who practice steadying their minds while facing the pressures of war. Imagine warfighters who practice steadying their minds in the face of great strife and despair. Imagine soldiers, trained in yoga, who are more likely to make the right call when the stakes were high. Imagine soldiers making hard calls on the front lines and being equipped with the tools of self-compassion and forgiveness to work through the reconciliation with moral injury. You might wonder how an hour at the gym's yoga class with a bunch of strangers would do that. The scientific literature on yoga for warfighters has spent more time focusing on treating pain and PTSD in veterans and not fully explored the questions of how yoga would fully enhance the skills of servicemembers. Ethnographic studies of the Nāyar clans of southern India suggest that there were warriors who used yogic tools as a fundamental part of their training and discipline.

Current scientific evidence suggests that two or three yoga classes per week can help back pain function, depressive and anxiety symptoms. Studies of yoga in active-duty populations have demonstrated that it is socially acceptable. Recent studies in Basic Training indicate that yoga can improve symptoms of sleep disorders and depression in new recruits. Yoga has been incorporated into integrated pain management programs at multiple military treatment facilities. According to the National Center for Health Statistics, yoga and meditation are two of the most popular complementary therapies used in the U.S.

I have both personally and professionally benefited from yoga as a soldier and ultimately a military medical practitioner. I have delivered yoga for studies of its affects in veterans, but my primary experience in both offering and receiving yoga has been individualized and relationship based. Before becoming a medical practitioner and after, I combined yoga, coaching, and community together. This integrated approach could be more powerful than any single method.

The research on yoga for the warfighter is not yet focused on optimizing performance. Instead of focusing on the current research, I offer an experience in three parts that explores how weaving yoga throughout a 20-year military career has added meaning and purpose to my life as a soldier, a medical professional, and a practitioner of therapeutic yoga.

What We Misunderstand About Yoga

One of the principal texts of yoga is the Bhagavad Gita, which chronicles the epic war of Mahabharata. The main character, Arjun is a warrior talking to Lord Krishna about the nature of war. As they are assembled along two sides of a battlefield, Arjun laments that he does not want to fight against his brothers, uncles, and cousins. He believes that the battle will kill so many senselessly and destroy the family and culture they had spent so much time cultivating. It is then that Lord Krishna says: "Indeed, for a warrior, there is no better engagement than fighting for upholding of righteousness." In this context, Arjun had a duty to fulfill in society. He was a soldier and to refuse to fight would be to turn away from his destiny. In Arjun's case, he was a soldier and could not be a soldier who refused to fight because it was not fulfilling his role in society.

There are many misconceptions about yoga. One of the most pervasive misunderstandings is that yoga is only about postures. Another is that yoga and meditation are completely different. Or that the postures need to be complicated or perfectly aligned for someone to benefit from the practice.

The foundation of yoga is its eight limbs outlined in the Yoga Sutras of Pantanjali.

They are:

1. *Yamas* – ethical guidelines
2. *Niyamas* – practices of character
3. *Asanas* – postures
4. *Pranayama* – breath control
5. *Pratyahara* – withdrawal of the senses
6. *Dharana* – concentration
7. *Dhyana* – meditation
8. *Samadhi* – enlightenment or bliss

The three limbs of yoga most familiar to the lay person are the third limb *asanas* (postures), the fourth limb *pranayama* (breathing) and the seventh limb *dhyana* (meditation). Some yoga instructors may also weave the experience of the fifth limb *pratyahara* (withdrawing of the senses) and the sixth limb *dharana* (concentration) while guiding people through postures. It is very common to attend a one-hour yoga class that focuses on postures with 1-2 minutes of deep breathing to help the student to or focus on their internal mind and body senses. The teacher may briefly guide the student into a practice of deep breathing or meditation at the end of class.

The first two limbs, yamas and niyamas have to do with principles of how we treat others and our own character development. The yamas include principles of kindness, truthfulness, not stealing, moderation, not being possessive. Niyamas include principles of character and explore concepts like cleanliness, contentment, discipline, contemplation and surrender to the divine. Some yogis might have reservations with the interpretation of the first yama as kindness and not ahimsa, which means non-harming. Soldiers are warfighters, not ascetics. It is more useful for them to operate from a principle of kindness and highest good, than a from an absolute principle of not harming anything.

For one to fully achieve their full capacity in the profession of arms, it's important to take the principles that will move people along to the next stage of development, not dogmatic perfection. Soldiers live on the threshold between the clashes of forces for more power. To defend what we value from harm, soldiers may need to do harm. The work of war is messy. The aspiration for perfection does not alleviate the need to defend imperfectly in the moment. Ahimsa is based on the concept that all beings are sacred. They are. Some beings have defenders, while others do not.

Part I:
From Hippie Girl to Military Yogi

I never should have been a soldier. My father was a post-Vietnam Marine who had nothing good to say about his experience. His message to me was always, get good grades and go to college. By 17, I was at Mills, a liberal arts women's college in the San Francisco Bay Area. The furthest career choice in my mind was the military. The furthest career choice from my mind was the military.

In 2003, the war in Iraq was scaling up. I just returned from a 10-month stint working in London after college and was at a local non-profit in Long Beach, California. My housemates and I tried to live a sustainable lifestyle full of daily yoga, raw vegan diets and modeling permaculture design principles. We practiced ashtanga yoga, which is typically a 90-minute series of the same yoga postures repeated every day. Ashtanga practice is designed to build physical and mental discipline. Although eventually, I would move towards other yoga traditions, ashtanga laid the foundation for regular yoga practice that I would carry forward with me for years to come.

Our home served as a hub for our organic food co-operative, where we grew backyard vegetables, respectfully foraged in our neighborhood, and promoted the local organic growers who shared our values. Our commitment to permaculture was pervasive in everything we did from grey water recycling and drip irrigation, to drought tolerant plants and lasagna gardening. We were about community. We even had an artist who rented tent space in our backyard. We were the type of community that one would expect to oppose America's involvement in the Iraq war.

We gathered at community potlucks to have meaningful discussions on world and national events. Our goal was not only to talk about the problems in the world, but also solutions. Conversations were broad, ranging from the morality and futility of the Iraqi war. The Iraqi war was tied to an homage about our dependence on fossil fuels. The dependence on fossil fuels was a cause of despair not only because of its link to the war, but also its link to climate change. As we discussed the need to move away from fossil fuels, someone would remark that the lasting ecological footprint of lithium in electric vehicles was almost as bad as fossil fuels. Another person would chime in on the benefits of biodiesel as a better alternative fuel. It became apparent that we were talking in circles. These solutions were hard. Nothing was absolute. But topics weren't always so heavy, attendees also shared delightful discoveries like the biological components of yerba mate and how you might prefer to drink it instead of coffee-- especially with a glass bombilla straw. Often, though, the conversations circled back to the war. It was what everyone was talking about.

At some point in these discussions, something started to feel off. It seemed that none of us fully understood what was going on in the war or the full implications of why our country might pursue that path. How could we? No one personally knew a soldier. No one was connected to anyone who dealt directly with foreign policy. What did we know other than what we were watching on CNN? Our conversations were heartfelt, but not fully informed. At some point, the conversations and our understanding felt lacking.

So, I walked into the Army Recruiter's office in Downtown Long Beach. I signed a 3-year contract to join the Army and find out.

I knew that my world would drastically change. It was a deliberate step away from my environment towards a space where I could reflect and observe. I imagined myself as a warrior monk, one who learned the craft of war, but approached warcraft with skilled mindfulness. My plan was to approach joining the Army as an anthropologist of sorts, immersing myself as a participant-observer. My goal was to glean insights about our country's role in foreign policy and truly understand what it meant to serve in the Iraq war. I did not fully appreciate how my former life would serve me in my new life. I would go to basic training, officer candidate school and the officer basic course. These steps were the beginning of truly understanding what it was like to be in the Army.

Part II:
From Basic Training to Yoga in the Heart of Iraq

During Basic Training, I was pleasantly surprised that before and after our morning workouts whether it was an obstacle course, a ruck march or a run, we did a little yoga. I don't think the drill sergeants thought of Conditioning Drills 1 and 2 as yoga. But, as they would stand on the platform shouting, "The Single-Leg Over!" and demonstrate the yoga position supine spinal twist, also known as supta masyendrasana, I was a little tickled. I was now getting paid to develop a habit that was difficult to sustain in civilian life: wake up before dawn, exercise and do yoga.

I finished Basic Training, Officer Candidate School, and the Officer Basic Course over the course of the next months. After school, I got orders to Fort Cavazos (formerly known as Fort Hood). Within 3 weeks of reporting, I was deployed to Operation Iraqi Freedom.

Not long after I arrived at our base in Iraq, a couple of soldiers from the military intelligence company approached me asking if I knew anyone who taught yoga. This was Fall of 2005 and yoga was getting more popular, but it was still a pretty niche request. I had some confidence in my abilities from my daily ashtanga practice at the co-op, but I was not certified. I told them, "I'm not an official yoga instructor, but I can show you what I know."

So, we brought our mats to the far reaches of the forward operating base and practiced. It was an hour of tapping into subtle physical sensation (pratyahara), breathing (pranayama) and allowing movement (asana) to flow until it was time to relax in Savasana. I now think of Savasana, the corpse pose, as a way to integrate all of the new movements we explored, a way to hear the sacred inner voice that all humans possess. It's a way to connect to our inner wisdom and to feel it in our bodies in stillness. But, at the time, I simply gave commands to lay on their backs with feet splayed, palms up, arms 45 degrees from the body, and breathing slowed way down. This was literally our moment of silence in the middle of the desert, midway between the Tigris and Euphrates rivers in an oasis of our own minds.

During our weekly practice, we cultivated a relationship with each other through mutual commitment to investigate our breath, our body sensations, and the serenity we felt when observing our bodies. The wisdom of our bodies communicated to us a sense of peace within each of us. Between us, there was also a sense of connection that permeated our practice. We relished in that sense of peace no matter what else was happening.

As a support platoon leader, I led some convoys, but much of my life was monotonous. I was not like the soldiers in Iskandaria, who at one point, lost a soldier every week. I was not like the soldiers in Diwaniyah who had to regularly negotiate the nuances of community engagements. I was not like the Cavalry Troops who had to pick up their friends' body parts off the main supply routes. I was not even like the support battalions who made so many supply runs that they lost one of their West Point 2LTs, Emily Perez. I had a charmed deployment in comparison: do physical training, go to the operations center, track convoys, monitor the radio, go to the motor pools, check maintenance paperwork, make sure supplies are ordered, listen to the first sergeant wax poetic, eat dinner, play dominoes at the cafe, and do it all again. It wasn't until loss came knocking on our door that we saw how valuable yoga was.

The first sergeant for the military intelligence company, Bobby Mendez was the type of guy who always found a way to connect to everyone around him. He intuited the needs of his soldiers and people felt safer knowing that he was around. My yoga students were his soldiers. Their teams were running convoys so frequently that First Sergeant Mendez decided to go out with his soldiers to boost morale. While he was out on a convoy, an enemy fighter hung an improvised explosive device from an overpass, and it killed him while he was riding in the gunner's hatch.

Like many who lost teammates in the war, we were numb. We went through shock, disbelief, sadness, bargaining, perhaps all of Elizabeth Kubler-Ross' stages of grief. When we went to the memorial ceremony for First Sergeant Mendez, we saw his boots, weapon and helmet arrayed like so many fallen soldiers. His memorial service was held in the exact location of our weekly yoga sessions. Then it hit me. There was something special about us memorializing him in the same space where we had been practicing yoga all the weeks before this day. We had built some equanimity within ourselves by practicing there. We had learned how to be ok when things were not ok. We learned how to listen to our inner wisdom. And maybe, in that moment of remembrance, we learned about the continuum, the connectedness between all soldiers.

Part III: Yoga as Medicine

In 2008, I deployed back to the same base in Iraq with a new team. My battalion commander helped me to get space in the gym to start teaching so more soldiers would know about yoga. After teaching yoga for a second year while deployed, I fully appreciated how important it was to be able to offer some mental respite for soldiers. I decided to get certified as a yoga instructor. During my 30 days of leave from Iraq, I went to the Kripalu Center for Yoga and Health and completed my 200-hour teacher training.

At Kripalu, I was able to dive deep into nourishing mind-body practices in a community of people who were all building new lives for themselves. I and the other students experienced a deep sense of listening to the body and watched the mind. The 30 days felt luxurious. I practiced yoga for 2-3 hours per day. The only foods and drinks available were healthy and delicious. I slept well. The environment was designed for health, for rest, for rejuvenation and preparing the body and the mind to receive new information and transform. It is only when writing this, some 15 years later, that I fully appreciate what elements were necessary to change my awareness down to the core.

It is only when reflecting that I realize what elements of my environment helped me to reach an optimal state. Kripalu created a structure that exuded order, created space, attuned to the sacred, was full of whole nutritious food, books, and conversations. It was a space designed for building connection and establishing comfort with ease. Kripalu helped me to realize how strikingly my environment can affect my mood. It still serves as an inspiration for what I can create for myself with every military move. If I paid attention and put in the work, I could deliberately create a space for myself to thrive.

On one of my first days of yoga teacher training at Kripalu, they did a skit of what goes on in the mind of the average yoga student while practicing. Three people took center stage in what seemed like a game of charades. One person was doing yoga postures, another person was jumping around, and the final person was just standing on the side watching it all happen.

The person doing the postures represented what we see people do in a yoga class. The person jumping around represented what our minds often do while we're in the postures, flitting from one thought to the next. The third person, standing and watching represented the higher self, what they referred to as witness consciousness. It was powerful to see all of the simultaneous actions that represented our mind, body and witness consciousness in a skit form. It felt true to my experience. Steven Pressfield, in The War of Art talks about what happens in our minds and bodies when we decide to practice any form of self-improvement – resistance. As soon as we focus on creating something bigger for ourselves, the mind starts to panic and looks for a way to escape.

At first, the mind resists yoga practice as well. The mind worries about the list of things we are not doing at the moment, it wonders if we are doing it right. The mind suspects a sinister outcome until we reassure the nervous system with more rhythmic with breathing.

In practicing breathing, moving into postures, concentrating, and withdrawing from the senses, we cultivated the experience of the witness. We noticed our thoughts as a part of our internal landscape, but not our entire internal landscape. We learned that our thoughts happened inside of us but were not us. It was also through yoga practice and mindful observation that we were able to be present with the fluctuations of the mind and notice that we have a witness observing it all. This awareness of the witness is a pathway to meditation, which is described by Nichala Joy Devi as an "inner flow of consciousness."

One of the key lessons from the time at Kripalu is how powerfully we could receive new ideas that change us for the better when our needs are supported. It was more than a one-hour class with strangers. Before we even arrived, a plan was designed for us to experience community, nourishing food, fulfilling physical and mental practices on a daily basis. It was the foundation of a lifestyle change. It allowed us to fully feel what is important, connect to our highest self, direct our executive function, and move forward with grace and ease. In Craig Bryan's book, Rethinking Suicide, he talks about the importance of building lives worth living to improve mental health. At Kripalu, by design, the community and environment held vital components that made life worth living.

Immediately after leaving Kripalu, I started the Interservice Physician Assistant (PA) Program in San Antonio. I went from the safe cocoon of Kripalu to the high stakes environment of PA school, where every lesson presented needed to be mastered. Any grade below a B on an exam could be the end of your education. The drumbeat of the program may have been "you must succeed," but for the students who were subject to high stakes consequences if the standards were not met, the message received was that you must not fail.

Yoga was my support along the way. I learned medicine, taught yoga, and supported local community gardens. Over the course of my didactic year, I started doing yoga in the back of the classroom so I could pay attention during 6-8 hours of science lectures daily and 2-3 exams per week. Yoga even became the focus of my master's thesis.

It wasn't until I arrived at my first assignment as a PA in South

Korea, did I fully appreciate how powerful yoga could be to take me from exhaustion to achievement. In Korea, I noticed that many of my soldiers were having sleep and other adjustment disorders from living in a new country. I assisted them with progressive relaxation, deep breathing and other mind-body practices that helped them to settle into their new roles. During the time I was working with my team and helping soldiers, I did not see how I was wearing myself down. About 3 months into my overseas rotation, I realized that I lost track of myself. I was a brand-new PA, who was still exhausted from the rigors of school and sent to practice in a remote area. The lingering sense of unease at being a brand new medical practitioner in a rural area and a large volume of patients left me spread thin.

My situation was compounded by difficult personnel transitions. Two other providers who worked in our clinic rotated back to the U.S. and my patient population tripled from 1000 to 3000 for three months. The stress was high, the stakes were high and the expectations I had for myself were high. At some point I was giving all I had, and I realized that I had no more to give. My self-care regimen was not consistent. I knew the tools to use. Alone and feeling disconnected, I found it difficult to sustain the nourishing practices I developed for myself during previous deployments, yoga training and even PA school.

By happenstance, I discovered this yoga studio in the Gangnam neighborhood of Seoul. Zen Yoga was a Korean application of yoga which was designed to be a comprehensive therapeutic program. It combined yoga classes, half-day workshops, one-on-one coaching, and massage. The impact of this was powerful. I saw how to implement yoga as therapy. The most meaningful components were: group practice (community), individual talk sessions (coaching and mentorship), individual massage sessions (healing), and home routines (discipline)

1. Group Practice: It was not a typical group practice class. Zen Yoga incorporated postures, breathing, withdrawal of the senses, concentration, and meditation, even meditation in motion. The classes were conducted in the context of staff emboding the yamas and niyamas in their community

interactions with each other and guests. People gathered after class to share food, drink and celebration. There was an authenticity with the practice that resonated within the organization. The power of authenticity and joy cannot be underestimated.

2. Individual talk sessions: One of the most powerful aspects of an individual talk session is deep listening from the wise guide. We don't talk about this enough. You don't have to be a therapist to listen to people and ask questions that can help put things in perspective. But the power of having someone act in this role of deeply listening can be profound.

3. Individual massage sessions: The abdominal massage was a curious process that I had not experienced before Zen Yoga or since. But, given that 90% of human serotonin is produced by the gut, this was a process that regularly shifted me into a state of relaxation, and it prepared me for the talk sessions with my yoga guide.

4. Home Routines: Each community member had a simple handout to use to track home yoga practices to help maintain the mind-body connection.

What I discovered during this process was that recommitting myself to yoga practice repeatedly with someone who was listening deeply to my concerns and offering support was something that I was missing from the public yoga classes I attended. Not since Kripalu had I felt so connected to myself and my practice. My yoga mentor also offered an opportunity to help me watch my thoughts. During this comprehensive process, my body was transformed. I was practicing on myself with the guidance of my yoga teachers. Ultimately, I was my own first client with remarkable results. Finding Korean Zen yoga helped me to transform from the edge of burnout to earning the Expert Field Medical Badge, which has a 13% success rate, running my first two marathons two weeks apart, and being hired as a Company Commander.

When I returned to the U.S., I pursued and accomplished a formal

Yoga Therapist certification. It was a process that included 500 hours of therapeutic yoga training as well as clinical mentorship hours with established Yoga Therapists. These mentors emphasized the same aspects of delivering care that I received in Korea.

Conclusion

The Army has recognized the need for holistic training and interventions for soldiers to reach optimal performance. It has even developed a Holistic Health and Fitness Manual to guide how physical therapists, occupational therapists, registered dieticians and athletic trainers can enhance the effectiveness of the warfighter. They train people in therapeutic relationships and support commanders in building cohesive teams.

What is missing is the training in the mind-body connection. Warfighters could also be offered healing Yoga Therapy practices in gyms, clinics and at home. Many military leaders know how to build cohesive teams and provide feedback. What's missing is that yoga can bridge the gap with helping soldiers feel cohesive not only with their teams, but with their inner wise guides. What's missing is popularizing the idea that warfighters can be fully integrated human beings. Soldiers, like all other people are capable of processing difficult emotions. They have the capacity to observe their thoughts and reframe. Community and mentorship are essential parts of the task. This takes practice, this takes discipline, this takes concentration and surrender to a higher power.

None of us fight wars alone. If we cultivate a mindful community, one that can integrate, meditate, and be prepared to fight when ready, perhaps it is one of the secret weapons we can provide for our warfighters for the next wars to come.

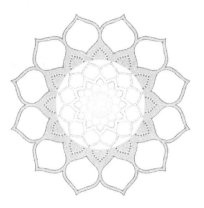

We're not going to tell you, "You have to do this one thing and you're going to feel better." No. We understand that it's a holistic perspective. You have to work on multiple layers of the human system. I'm excited to see things like pain research and brain research support what we're already doing.

~Amy, C-IAYT

A Sherpa's Perspective of Yoga Therapy
Banton Dyer, CPT, C-IAYT

What is the hardest thing to accomplish in your life if you are already a billionaire, a well-known socialite, a top psychiatrist, or a retired international spy? It's really the same thing that was so hard for me when I was a young, abused, and neglected 16-year-old boy who only wanted to learn how to beat people up. The lesson is deceptively simple but incredibly challenging: Relaxing enough to let go of the driver's wheel of your life, to genuinely rest, to develop the insight and see what is really going on in front of you, using disciplines like martial arts and yoga.

To be good at fighting, I had to learn this. To be good at recovering from a stroke, overcoming suicidal depression, or facing the fathomless decrepity of old age, my clients had to learn this. Whether it took them one session or 20 years, I was there for them, like a Sherpa, guiding them step by step. In this chapter, we'll delve into why this simple task is so hard and yet so easy, why it's worth the work, and how the role of a 'Sherpa'—a Yoga Therapist—becomes indispensable in this transformative journey.

What is this? Relaxing enough to let go of the driver's wheel of your life. Relaxing enough to actually go into a deep restful sleep. Relaxing enough to practice martial arts or yoga effectively. So that you can live the life you want to live and live well.

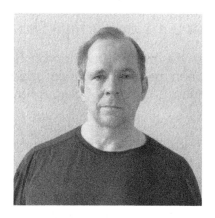

Banton Dyer is sought after for his hard core, yet heart-centered guidance, and is known for helping you find healthy ways to cultivate your focus and vitality.

Relying on his background in Yoga Therapy, physical training, and martial arts, Banton supports you to transform your life as you become the healthy vibrant individual you know you can become.

Over the past 35 years Banton has worked with people with different backgrounds, from people on their last dollar all the way to billionaires. His clients have come to expect nothing but the highest level of care and compassion from him — even when he is challenging them to take their next best step in difficult times.

Whether your challenges are in board rooms, at home or on the street, Banton knows how to get to the heart of your concerns and apply a personalized and well-honed approach to helping you be successful.

His strength lies in having overcome life's most challenging situations himself and the ability to empathetically help others to overcome overwhelming trials in their lives. He has a deep passion for helping people to find their own way to physical and emotional restoration, no matter how busy or difficult their life, so that they can experience the joy of being supported in what they love or desire to do most.

What is a Yoga Therapy Sherpa?

Well, it's just my way of explaining my approach to teaching. The only difference between me and the typical yoga teacher is education and experience, and that I always have my client's back.

The sherpa is not a guru. The Sherpa is an educated expert, skilled and knowledgeable, the guide, who brings the ancient practices into modern times, so they become relevant and relatable. There is a softness to the Sherpa's guidance; understanding, listening, relatable, person to person. To me, the Yoga Therapist is the Sherpa, who is needed now.

How do you define Yoga Therapy?

It's taking the knowledge of yoga and the heart of yoga, and putting it into western healthcare. Being an advocate for the client. And other times, giving them truly traditional work, like breathwork, or something of that nature that's transformative.

What is sacred yoga to you?

The sacred part would be the heart in the sense of caring about the client. Looking at them as Atma, or soul, that's divine no matter what they have going on.

What does the future of Yoga Therapy look like?

I believe it will become more mainstream and more integrated with healthcare. And also separate from healthcare, accessible for people that may not have the money for psychiatric care or something like that, because one of the most powerful areas that yoga handles is the mind.

What would you say to someone who is looking at Yoga Therapy and trying to find the right Yoga Therapist?

What I wish for you is to be inspired and directed or guided into your own path into some type of journey with God.

What I wish for you is to see a glimpse of the way I work. So that I might help you get inspired to have some type of physical growth, emotional growth, or spiritual growth.

You will know that you have found the right person when you feel safe and inspired.

How do we open to receive?

Well my experience has been that if you want to improve or grow in life, many times part of it is painful. And part of it is learning to transform the ego, so that we can see the truth of our behaviors. Our belief structure is not what we thought it was. We have to let go of that. And that's usually not fun. When you let go of the grip of the ego, you will be able to receive deeply and feel your spirit uplifted in many ways.

What do you want people to remember?

I think there's way too much emphasis on the physicality of a lot of the yoga that's out there, instead of what it was really about was meditation, and listening to God/Higher Power or finding your own self. It's the Divine Source - some means of connecting to a higher power. Something to remind you of your own divinity and everybody else's. To me, yoga is more like a practice that allows you to develop and maintain a disciplined mind.

The yoga sutras tell you that the whirlwinds of the mind are a means to unhappiness. Your ability to focus your mind where you want it helps you to keep your mind and emotions steady and smooth. This leads to feelings of deep peace, joy and gratitude.

What do you like best about being a Yoga Therapist?

That I get to help others. I was a Yoga Therapist way before I even got into Yoga Therapy, because I was doing this stuff with martial arts and it was doing something similar. And I was like, Oh, well, y'all are doing what I do. But I'm learning ways to do it more organized, more effectively for more people. I also get to help people find their own way of helping themselves.

Here's a story from a Vedic priest to explain it: There's this house, and in one room you have people that have had a green light bulb, and they screw the light bulb into the lamp and they pray and meditate with God's green light. In another room, they have a red light bulb, and they screwed it into a lamp and God is red. And then they both get in the hallways and they get to talking. And it's like, "No, God's green guys. Really!" No God is red" And then they'll tear each other's eyes out and kill each other over who is right, instead of realizing that God is the source of the electricity that's lighting the light bulb. It's just different interpretations of God.

God is all about love. Loving yourself, loving your neighbor, not judgment. And that's what yoga is about.

Can you give us some examples
of your own journey and use of Yoga Therapy?

I turned to Martial Arts to beat people up, but surprisingly got a sense of silence and serenity in the war zone of my mind. This was the beginning of my inner and outer journey, which has brought me to where I am today, leading others in their own journey through Yoga Therapy. Yoga came into my life, soon afterwards which helped me to go even deeper. When I was learning yoga I noticed the similarities between its core tenets and martial arts.

When I took the next steps into Yoga Therapy that is where I began healing at a deeper level of my emotions and my soul. This was where I was given assignments that were specifically for me - well beyond asanas, the physical postures, I learned meditation, breathing and yoga philosophy including such tenants as Ahimsa, non-violence to others, and maybe most importantly for me, non-violence to self.

Seeing the different modalities teaching the same principles, helped convince myself of the truth of these teachings. This gave me more confidence in myself and trust in utilizing these practices. When I later went through my divorce, I was at an all-time low emotionally and physically.

In my darkest days, particularly during my divorce, I felt lost and disconnected. It was Yoga Therapy that helped me find my center again. The practice was like a lighthouse guiding me through the stormy waters of my own life.

Yoga was my trusted refuge. I integrated the growth experiences I got from martial arts into my approach and personal use of Yoga Therapy practice, and found the results to be very powerful. Especially when I integrated the yoga practice of ahimsa (non-violence), I was able to feel a sense of self-love and a glimpse of experiencing divinity for the first time despite the challenges I was facing in my contentious, difficult, challenging, soul tearing divorce.

Eventually through Yoga Therapy and prayer, I was able to see first the divinity in my own self. Later and with even more difficulty I was able to see the divinity in my ex-wife. This allowed me to let go of the past experiences and forgive her, so that I could move on with my life in a healthy and productive way.

And now if I have difficulty or resentment with someone, not only do I use prayer, I look to see the divinity in that person, and remind myself of my own divinity. Just as a Sherpa must be experienced climbing the mountain, my Yoga Therapy is informed by my experiences and use of it. Mere intellectual knowledge of these practices won't get you very far. It gets you no trust with your clients and you need to be able to trust your Sherpa to survive and thrive.

Tell us about some of the types of clients you have and how you work with them.

While immediate relief might be the primary goal for many, the unseen benefits—emotional balance, spiritual growth, and even improved relationships—are just as critical.

A retired international spy, trained to endure high levels of stress, came to me seeking relief from lung issues. He wanted quick results. I tried to explain that yoga is not like taking a pill. Though you can experience some immediate changes, deep healing of emotional, mental and physical issues will take time. You can't climb the mountain the day you decide you want to. You have to do the work. The Sherpa, like the Yoga Therapist, is the guide. You have to build your own muscles, do your inner work and be prepared to move forward in your journey.

Sometimes my role is telling people what they don't want to hear. However, this allows them to see clearly and then decide for themselves when they are ready to put in the work. Eventually this person did get better, because they finally realized they had to work – work to relax and do practices that aren't necessarily as thrilling as international spy work, but ultimately, thrilling in a different and more profound way.

The commercial world might want you to believe in instant miracles, but the truth, as this client's journey showed, is that authentic Yoga Therapy requires patience and commitment.

One billionaire client, a titan in the energy industry, came to me initially seeking ways to manage stress and to relax. Despite having the world at her fingertips, she found it impossible to simply relax. The first few sessions involved not advanced postures but merely learning to breathe deeply. As simple as this sounds, I needed to be patient with her. In the fast-paced business environment in which she thrived, slowing down to breathe was completely foreign. As part of the journey I the Sherpa also led her to reducing physical pain and stabilizing her joints especially to relieve her knee pain. Over time, she found herself more focused, less reactive in high-stakes board meetings, and reported feeling genuinely relaxed for the first time in years.

One of my most memorable experiences involved a young stroke survivor. Doctors had told him he'd never regain full motor skills, let alone walk. He was having none of that. At first, he wanted me to help him run even though he was still in a wheelchair. As the sherpa, I had to explain the path required for him to develop safe and effective walking first. Under my guidance he came to understand that climbing the mountain is a marathon not a sprint. We worked together over five years, combining Yoga Therapy with his medical treatments. Today, he's walking, having regained half of his mobility and cherishes the simple joys of life. He is the hardest working client I have ever had. Importantly he learned to listen to me when I told him to take it easy.

In another example of less is more, a top psychologist whom I worked with was repeatedly experiencing burn-out. Like a Sherpa showing the road map, I pointed out how he was burning the candle at both ends and that though he was working hard he was not working optimally. Again, my honesty with him gained his trust and though it took time, with my guidance, instead of intellectualizing the problem, he became more aware of what was happening in a way he could make changes. This was accomplished primarily through breathing and meditative techniques and applied yoga philosophy.

One of the things I say is though some of these practices are simple, you have to be doing them daily, or regularly at least. If you don't do them, they don't work. When you do them as prescribed by your Yoga Therapist, they work!

One client, a surgeon, was going through a difficult time with his wife, which created a lot of anxiety and uncertainty in his life. Before he was good at partitioning his personal life and his professional life. He got to a point where it was just too overwhelming and he sought my advice. So I said, well, nobody's gonna follow you into the bathroom before surgery. So go in there, sit down. Take a few breaths to breathe for a while and do this until you can calm your mind. He reported back that this simple practice made him feel calmer and able to focus at work as he did in the past. And that's good news! No one wants a distracted surgeon.

I remember a socialite who was my client. Many of my clients spent decades hopping from one wellness fad to another. Sometimes when they come to me, in their mind Yoga Therapy is their last resort. They knew I was always being honest with them. They knew I had their back. They finally would commit to long-term work because they knew they could trust me. They gained newfound stability and groundedness from which they could heal and thrive or improve in ways that they would have never expected simply because they finally made the commitment.

This is why it's worth the work; it's not just about symptom relief, but about deep, transformative change that permeates every aspect of life. One of the most profound realizations I've had is that everything is interconnected. This philosophy can turn a session of simple breathing exercises into a deeply transformative experience.

Conclusion

In summary, the kinds of clients I attract tend to have a lot of different kinds of pain or dysfunction or both. I also work with people who are athletes or want to be athletes and they want to improve their performance. Most are working at a high level in their career or personal life, and they tend to be leaders in their communities. I help bring them into balance so that physically, mentally and emotionally they are achieving and finding success in their leisure hours, and will have the fortitude to keep going, doing the things they love for the long run in their personal and spiritual lives as well. I tell them, "We do this _____, so that you can do that_____" Insert here what you want to do most, (i.e. fly fishing, pick up your grandkids, travel, ride elephants...) and then I fill in the first apart with the Yoga Therapy techniques I have you practice to get the results you desire..

In the beginning of my journey into adulthood, I began wanting to be better at violence and found myself instead embracing non-violence and relaxing into a situation in order to get the things I always had wanted then and now; Spiritual connection to God, sense of serenity, feeling good in my body and self-love.

In preserving the sacred future of Yoga Therapy, the role of the Yoga Therapist is not just as an instructor but as a guide, a confidant, and above all, a Sherpa individually guiding his flock through the treacherous terrains of modern wellness.

Whether you are a high achieving billionaire or a young, abused individual, the task remains the same: learning to relax deeply, so that you can listen to your inner self and then have the power to do whatever is asked of you. Relaxing is a universal challenge but also the key to mastering various aspects of life. The Sherpa's job is not just guiding you but making sure you can carry yourself forward into whatever life throws your way.

OM Mantra Meditation for You

I want to leave you with a gift of a simple practice that has carried me through many times when I was having difficulty finding a quiet place in my mind. I think of this kind of meditation as if you were on a boat out on the sea where the water is really choppy. Instead of trying to make the water perfectly calm, you just throw an anchor down. You still bob around with the water, but the anchor keeps you in place.

One woman I worked with would practice this particular meditation during her flight layovers. There is no excuse for not finding five minutes. Stay in the bathroom for 5 extra minutes if needed. Very rapidly you will want to do it because it will become obvious that it is something you need and now want to do because you are feeling so much better.

This mantra meditation is something that I pick for students when they are having a hard time meditating. All you have to do is repeat the mantra over and over again. It doesn't matter if you think of other things. You just keep repeating the mantra.

OM Mantra Meditation Instructions

Say the word OM out loud and repeat it over and over again (which by the way this particular single word mantra, has been scientifically studied and found to be highly effective).

Gradually repeat more and more softly.

Then work to have it just inside your head, so you are mentally repeating the word OM.

Then the idea is to even practice saying OM quieter and quieter in your mind.

I find it beneficial to imagine a large gong vibrating and making the OM sound with me in my mind. Try to imagine feeling the vibrations of the gong as if your own OM mantra practice is also vibrating within you.

Do not be concerned if your mind starts thinking of other things and is distracted. Just bring it back to repeating OM. There is no way to do this wrong. The only wrong thing is to not do it at all. In fact I have found that many times that I had so many things going on in my mind I didn't feel I was "meditating", were actually the times I benefited the most. My mind was more clear and grounded throughout the rest of the day or with my evening practice, I slept better.

I recommend that you start out with 5 minutes in the morning and 5 minutes in the evening. Then work up to 20 minutes of each.

If you would like to hear me lead you through these instructions and guide you: https://www.trainingwithbanton.com/

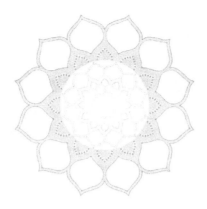

It's about informing Yoga Therapists and yoga teachers from both an Eastern perspective and a Western perspective. I think of ourselves as educators, as yogis, yoginis and Yoga Therapists.

~Richard, C-IAYT

The Pain That Became a Separate Reality

Nicole DeAvilla,
E-RYT500, RPYT, RCYT, C-IAYT

I became a yoga teacher because my back hurt. At the height of my back problems, I had thoracic (upper back) pain, sciatica pain radiating down my legs, and pinched nerves that kept me from turning my head in a normal fashion.

I felt an intensive yoga program would help. It did, and one important side effect was that I learned to meditate, which changed my life permanently for the better. But in addition to the usual difficulties of a beginning meditator, sitting was the worst position for my back pain.

A loss of body consciousness

One day I was determined to try my best to go deeper in meditation and transcend the pain. I remembered being told that visualizing a saint's eyes was a powerful technique for meditation.

At that time, I knew little about saints. However, I had read Swami Kriyananda's book, *The Path*, so I decided to look at his cover photo. I closed my eyes and, with all my will power, focused on his eyes.

It was tough going. The back cried out as usual for attention. Eventually, to my amazement and enjoyment, I was able to transcend the pain! Through the strong concentration, I experienced a loss of body consciousness. To be free of pain, even for a short time, was a wonderful and expansive feeling.

The most intense back pain ever

More than twenty years had passed since that experience. Gradually, through yoga and other techniques, my back healed.

However, I re-injured it. Applying all the healing techniques I knew, within a few weeks I managed to reduce the pain to a slight twinge.

Then one night I was up late working on a writing assignment. My five-year-old daughter was having trouble going to sleep and had climbed into bed with her father. Both my daughter and husband were asleep when I went to pick her up and return her to her room, as I have done many times.

This time, however, I forgot all about the body mechanics I had learned over the past twenty years. I reached toward the middle of the bed and picked her straight up.

Fortunately, she was only a few inches above the bed when my back "went out" and I dropped her. The pain was more intense than any back pain I had ever felt. I let out a sound that woke both my daughter and husband, and somehow came down onto the floor, where I lay on my back next to the bed, with my knees bent.

With this pain I knew I needed help

I focused immediately on deep diaphragmatic breathing— breathing deeply into the belly and blowing out the pain with my exhalations. My husband and daughter rushed to help me. I asked them not to touch me.

Normally I take medication only as a last resort. However, without much hesitation, I asked for Ibuprofen. With this pain I knew I needed help. Then I asked my husband if he would gently cover me with a blanket. I convinced him and my daughter (in between deep breathing) to go to bed, that I could take care of myself.

The spasms were intense. I had to use my breath just to maintain the pain at the current level. If I even attempted a therapeutic pelvic tilt, the spasms would deepen and increase.

There was no reason not to still be joyful

As I lay there working with the breath and consciously trying to relax the spasms, I automatically went into my usual practice of mentally chanting, "I love you God." I focused at the spiritual eye and invoked Yogananda and Divine Mother's presence.

Shifting into a more God-conscious state made me recall that I had been feeling very joyful before my back went out. I reflected that, though I was in pain, I was grateful for many things in my life and that there was no reason not to still be joyful.

I then started mentally chanting one of my other personal mantras, "joy, joy, joy"— all the while breathing deeply to control the pain. Chanting "joy" reminded me that joy was still part of my core being.

Somehow I knew I had a choice: I could feel sorry for myself (poor me!), and worried about the possibility of a long and difficult rehabilitation. Or I could stay in the present moment, get back to my center, and experience joy. I chose joy.

Two separate and distinct realities

It wasn't a matter of pretending that the pain did not exist. In fact, I needed to focus part of my attention on the deep breathing to keep the pain from intensifying and spreading.

Gradually, however, despite the pain (and the need to focus on it), my awareness of joy expanded. Before long I was feeling great joy. The pain was as intense as ever. But I was experiencing two separate and distinct realities: pain and joy.

It was a revelation that I could experience such a depth of joy and still be aware of physical pain. I had always assumed that saints who remained joyful despite great physical trials had transcended body consciousness in ecstasy.

But I recalled something I had read about St. Teresa of Avila.

When not in ecstasy, she often experienced great physical pain. However, in her joyful devotion to the work Christ had given her, she was only partially aware of it. Not all saints with serious physical ailments, I began to realize as I lay on the floor, lived in a constant state of ecstatic communion. Their joy in God was so intense, however, that physical pain simply did not matter.

When the spasms became less intense, I was able to move into a therapeutic pelvic tilt. After half an hour of deep breathing and gentle pelvic tilts, I was able to get up. I placed pillows under my knees—and, covering myself with blankets from the bed— went to sleep on the floor.

I am deeply grateful

The physical healing took a while. I slept on my back on the floor with my legs over a padded bench for almost a week. For several weeks I asked both my daughter and seven-year- old son to be very careful with me— too forceful a hug could be extremely painful.

As I applied my knowledge of therapeutic yoga and other techniques, I tried to focus on God, Guru, and the joy within. Whenever I became focused and centered, I once again experienced joy.

I am deeply grateful for the blessing of the pain that was not transcended but became a separate reality. It has helped me see that the goal of life is not necessarily to remove or even transcend life's difficulties, but to live in joy regardless of the ups and downs.

As I live this way, the more things tend to work out for the best. Challenges still come but as I live more deeply from my center in God, I am able to handle them more gracefully.

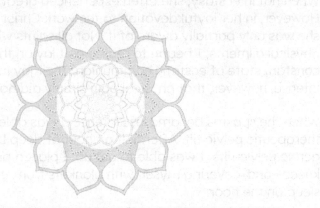

Yoga Therapy is part of yoga. Yoga is much broader than healthcare. We always say, keep the "yoga" in Yoga Therapy. Yoga Therapy is not just about fixing your back. It's a doorway to lots of things.

~ John, C-IAYT

The Lesson of the Smoke Detector

Nicole DeAvilla,
E-RYT500, RPYT, RCYT, C-IAYT

I taught yoga and meditation in a beautiful studio complete with an altar, weekly fresh flowers arrangements by a Japanese master, and lovely natural light from the skylights in the curved ceiling. Except for occasional bursts of low-level noise from the bike shop on one side, and the restaurant on the other, the environment is "perfect"—beautiful, uplifting, and quiet.

A loud piercing sound

One morning, as I was preparing my class for deep relaxation and guided meditation, we were suddenly jarred by the loud piercing sound of a smoke detector announcing that its battery was low. The offending object was attached to the wall near the two story high ceiling and there was no way I could disarm it.

Hoping for the best, I assured my students that "it was just a battery problem" and nothing to be concerned about. But after a few minutes it went off again, and thereafter continued to beep intermittently.

Tensed for flight of fight!

Imagine lying comfortably in deep relaxation, a pillow under your head or a bolster under your knees for maximum comfort, mind and body prepared to relax and renew after an invigorating morning class of Ananda Yoga. You hear the words "Bones, muscles, movement, I surrender now; anxiety, elation, depression, churning thoughts, all these I give into the hands of Peace." (Ananda Yoga™ Affirmation)

You are drifting into a state of deep relaxation and then WHAM! a loud, piercing, grating sound, designed to awaken people out of their deepest slumber, jolts you back into your body, now tensed for flight or fight!

This gives some idea of what I was up against. If the class was to continue, I needed to find a solution—quickly.

My prayer is answered

Swami Kriyananda suggests that mentally placing a blue cross of light over a phone, door, or person can deflect negative energy, so I tried it. Not surprisingly, it didn't work. There was nothing negative about the noise; it was a neutral event. I was the one who was becoming negative.

I also prayed feebly for the beeping to stop—"feebly" because I was annoyed and distracted, not at all focused and concentrated. Still, feeble as it was, I think my prayer was answered.

Suddenly I had the thought not to reject the sound but to incorporate it into the deep relaxation and guided meditation. In the spirit of embracing the situation, I asked the class to actively listen for the sound of the alarm, and to count each beep, giving each a number: one, two, three, etc. This brought smiles to their faces.

No longer tensing against it

They began to count silently and I practiced with them. The beeping continued intermittently but we were no longer tensing against it while also trying to relax. We were now receptive, ready to name it, and to organize it with numbers.

While counting the beeps, we were also counting our breaths— inhale 4, hold 7, exhale 8. We were experimenting with a new type of measured breathing that required more concentration than the usual even count breathing (inhale 8, hold 8, exhale 8).

More focused on the present

For all of us, the extra effort of counting the beeps and our breaths had the effect of keeping our thoughts focused and in the present moment. Calmly centered, we continued counting the beeps as we sat for the guided meditation.

Later I recalled Swami Kriyananda's description of being at the dentist's and choosing to go through the procedure without pain medication. He tolerated the pain by remaining centered in the spine and breath. When the pain became too intense to ignore, he would focus on the pain and go to the center of it. At the center, the pain disappeared.

We were not able to go deeply enough into the sounds to banish them from our consciousness, but we entered into them deeply enough to completely transcend our frustration. What we had been dreading and bracing against was no longer a concern—it simply was.

A life lesson in calm acceptance

At the end of the guided meditation, the students had peaceful and happy expressions. We all agreed that bringing the sound of the smoke detector into our meditation had brought a deeper than usual experience. It was a life lesson in calmly accepting the things over which we have no control, and not letting them rob us of our peace.

Out in the waiting room we could still hear the beeping of the alarm, but the sound no longer bothered us. Before leaving, however, one student said, "You will ask the management to fix it won't you?"

After all, keeping your peace means accepting what you can't change and also acting to change what you can!

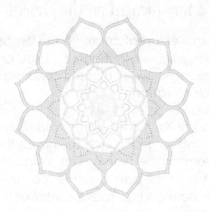

IAYT is the most sense of family that I've found. I've never been to yoga conferences before where there's been such a sense of comradery, support, authenticity and love. We're holding each other up with what we're bringing out into the world while also having a sense of quality to the standards of what we're bringing. If that's something that you believe in, and you want to find a yogic home, I think IAYT is top notch.

~Stephanie L, C-IAYT

Dharma and the Present

Nicole DeAvilla,
E-RYT500, RPYT, RCYT, C-IAYT

Dharma: Your life purpose. Each of us is born with a calling, a right way of living. Each person's dharma is unique. To fully realize ourselves, and best serve others, we need to act in alignment with our dharma.

When you do not live according to your dharma, whether through circumstances real or self-imposed, or out of lack of knowledge, then you will never truly be happy let alone fulfilled.

It is tempting during chaotic times in the world, in our personal circumstances or both, to sit back and wait it out before taking bold action. We wait, maybe too long, before launching into a new phase of life or taking on what we truly know is our soul's calling.

The folly is that if we do not act, if we do not move forward - even when we are uncertain of the path - our own life will become more chaotic not less and our ability to deal with outside chaos will also diminish.

The good news is that you do not have to do this alone. Even though we each have a unique calling, we can grow and move together. We can learn from each other. We can be in community to support and bolster and fortify each other for those times when we do have to occasionally walk alone.

Dharma

I woke up. The sky was orange, a dark ominous orange. There was no sun. It was wrong. So wrong. Fires had been burning all across California and air quality was often hazardous. The pandemic was still raging. The desire to find safe ways to connect in person was strong.

I had one of my first group events in over a year scheduled for this day, on this foreboding, dark burnt orange day. It wasn't long before the leader of our event sent out an email. She wrote: "Sadly, we have to cancel today due to unprecedented darkness (what?!) I had backup plans for pandemics and fires, but total darkness in the redwoods has stumped me a bit. It's simply too dark in the retreat location for us to have a good experience."

Darkness. Chaos. Division. War. Pandemic, Fires, Floods... I never used to believe the predictions.

My revered teacher Swami Kriyananda often spoke of the great yoga Master, our guru, Paramhansa Yogananda's predictions made many decades earlier. It was always in the background of my consciousness. Predictions of turmoil, food shortages, supply change issues, war - maybe World War 3 - were never given to scare, cause fear, division or create a following.

These predictions were given so that we could be prepared, personally empowered and be the ones who were bearing the light, bringing hope and leading the world in our own unique ways into a new era, a more peaceful, spiritual time at the other end of the chaos.

As time unfolded I sometimes thought - this must be it. We are here... Alas those were just preludes. As we approach the apogee of the turmoil, the divisions, war and chaos, simultaneously there is no end in sight and the comfort of validation that there is not an end, but a new better way of being.

I am understanding more clearly. I am seeing my role more clearly. I didn't think I had a role of any significance. I am letting go. I am letting go of old thought patterns. I am letting go of ways that no longer serve me or perhaps never served me. Thus I am more powerfully serving others.

Now I understand, more than ever I need to tune in to and rely on the divine presence and guidance of my spiritual lineage. I keep hearing the silent whisper, "Do more Kriyas. Do more Kriyas." In other words, meditate deeply as taught by my guru, dive into my chakras and the cosmic sound of AUM; be divinely connected. "Do more Kriyas" is the answer to all of my big questions.

When I do more Kriyas, more meditation and tuning inward and aligning to the divine, the result is what I need to do, what I need to let go of, and the strength and energy to do it, comes. When I do my inner work, I find that which needs to happen, unfolds almost seemingly without effort, almost magically.

I have been encouraging my clients and students to do their inner work too. To my surprise, I am finding myself on fire preaching this message of how to be prepared, be ready and be a shining light for others - all in their own unique ways, more often. I also guide them in the how - How to be more you! How to fulfill your dharma. If you don't - if you decide to attempt to sit on the sidelines and watch, I am sorry. You will get knocked down. Knocked to your knees. And they get it. They feel it. They know it.

This is how all of us find our pure potential - through introspection, guidance and taking action. Doing the little things in life, so that we are ready for the big ones, is a daily practice. We need to do our dharma, the work we are meant to do in this life. Not someone else's. And we need to do it now. It is the difference between riding the wave and being crushed by it.

This apogee, this grand terrible time predicted by many religions, masters and prophets, is not the end of the world.

It is not the end of the world. It is the end of old ways of living in this world. We can either let go of the old ways – dogmatism, institutionalism, – a whole bunch of isms! – or we can try to hold onto them and get whipped around, pummeled and thrown like a surfer being harshly thrown to the hard sand surface at the bottom of the ocean.

If we keep trying to ride the waves – and they are getting faster, bigger, more beautiful and more dangerous – in old ways and in ways that belong to other people, not our new ways, it will happen again. And again. How many times do you want to be tossed to the bottom of the ocean?

How do we navigate this? How do we catch the big beautiful wave that will bring us thrillingly to the warm beach of soft sand safely and soundly? And be ready to do it again. And again. With energy, with grace, with strength and with love.

We can't hold onto our old ways, to others' old ways. We can't sit back choosing to sit this one out as we drink lemonade and paddle about on our backs relaxing under a warm salty sun in a calm blue ocean. If you try to do this, you will not see the next wave coming – and it will knock you to your knees (at best).

So how do we do this? Step by step. Day by day. It starts with what you feed your mind when you first wake up in the morning. It starts with being you, more, more you. Let me explain.

The way I wake up most of the time in the morning when I am on my A game, is steeped in modern science, ancient wisdom and spirituality. It hasn't always been that way. My proclivity to burning the candles at both ends has not served me well. Sometimes it may have seemed that I was getting more done, having more fun by staying up late socializing and I frequently had deadlines to meet, so I felt I had no choice.

I used to think that I needed more hours in the day – that would solve so many of my problems! In my early twenties I was racked with pain. The pain brought me to yoga, some 40 years ago. One of the side effects I experienced with yoga was perspective. I eventually realized that if I was given more hours in the day, I would commit myself to more projects and people.

Still burning the candles at both ends has been an addiction for me, buried deep within my psyche it has been hard for me to break the cycle.

I read that my guru, Paramhansa Yogananda once said: routinize your life.

It was a terrifying, difficult statement for me to read! I was routineless! Hopelessly so, I thought. At the time I was pregnant with my first child. I knew babies and children thrive with good routines. I vowed to at least create routines for them.

And I must say, I did fairly well with that! My kids, young adults now, have many good routines under their belts — and do better with them than I. Little by little I began to create some of my own routines, and have been reasonably consistent with them.

Years later I took a Strengths test. It showed my bottom, very last, strength is Consistency. When I saw that, I knew the test was accurate! I figure if I can create routines, anyone can!

Here is the good news. You don't have to be perfect with your routines, your daily habits. I'm not!

Some routines you will want to work toward setting them in stone, even if your stone feels more like concrete that is taking years to dry! Your routines will evolve as you evolve. To begin, choose low hanging fruit - find the easiest routines or habits for you to add into your current lifestyle.

After you have had some success, you might want to give more focus on habits that will be the most impactful for your health and well being. Those can help build a solid foundation for your other routines and activities. This is the foundation you need to do your dharma consistently, with energy and joy.

Why build routines and create new habits? If you want something other than what you have now in your life, whether that be more energy, better health, better relationships, better finances, more abundance, peace of mind, deeper connection to your dharma... you get the idea. You will need new habits and ways of doing things. The old ways clearly won't work - or you would have these things now.

For example, I had joint pain. The pain was often debilitating and it kept me from fully doing my work, my dharma. I had to change my diet and use natural supplements. It took awhile for me to be consistent with both of these. Once I developed new eating habits and some consistency in taking my supplements, I stopped having chronic joint pain. I had more energy and focus to do my life's calling.

Of course all of that pain has taught me much - I have had acute and chronic pain in every major joint in my body and some not so major! Maybe that is why I get referrals to work with the tough cases, people for whom traditional health care doesn't work so well.

If I don't do these things, if I fail to care for myself, to do my inward practices, at best I get distracted from doing my dharma. At worst I am unable to do my dharma -- and that is a miserable place to be.

Learning something new can be a challenge. One of my coaching clients, was averse to moving more of his business online. I knew his goals, his abilities and his dharma and felt the timing was right. So I insisted that he learn.

By the time the Covid Pandemic hit and nearly everyone was forced to do business online, he was a pro at it. He made a smooth transition with his clients. He continued to move froward with his work, his dharma. He saw his colleagues struggling and too many of them had to quit or barely get by.

A little preparation - even if it is hard, and feels unnatural at first can go along way. We need to be preparing ourselves now.

So what does all of this have to do with the prophecies of doom and gloom and the promise of better times ahead of eons of peace and deeper spiritual lives? I have a calling – just as you do. We all do. In order to do my dharma, I need to be healthy, well rested and waking up in my A game. Ready to ride the ever growing, ever more frequent waves of change and challenge.

I need to be strong enough and sharp enough to help others too. Because that is my dharma. Your dharma may call you in a different direction, to do different things. I can assure you however, that it is not going to lead you to old ways, ways that soon won't work anymore – even if they seemed to work in the past.

Growing up I found I had natural talent and natural success in many things. Mind you this was not without many, many difficult challenges like 5 major surgeries before the age of 18 to name one. I also love learning. As I got older, I learned and studied more in the areas where I wanted success. The more I studied, the more I learned the more I was the good student, the less success I had.

It has taken effort and time to reflect, realize who I really am, what makes me tick, what is unique to me. I need to do more Kriyas and be open to what my divine messages are. I need to start being more like my old self in many ways. I need to be more me, with better habits!

Asking for help isn't always easy, especially for women. I have one client whom I have worked with off and on for many years now. There have been times when I check in with her and find that she has been struggling for some time with health or work issues - they often go hand-in-hand don't they? At that point she invites me in. Her joy when she feels the constriction of confusion, self-doubt and being relentlessly hard on herself, come off like a butterfly finally ready to fly and drink the sweet nectar of life, is infectious.

Please don't wait. If you need help coming out of your cocoon, act now! A butterfly set free can fly upwards to safety and the support of tall trees when the waves of life grow large and raging, unlike the cocoon who will be trapped and stuck.

Now I am not an actual surfer. I can't even say I am a swimmer, though I can swim. Even so the image of you, me and many others beautifully adorned in bright colored wetsuits to match our individuality, riding a super wave, a powerful wave awesome, beautiful and potentially deadly, and making it thrillingly and joyfully back to a sandy smooth beach keeps coming to my mind.

Being a good surfer, takes practice and good daily habits. You don't just wake up one day and decide you can surf big waves. You might need to get in better shape first, take swim lessons in the ocean, work on your balance and start with small waves on a calm day.

That's where good daily habits comes in to play. Life is always throwing curve balls. We need to be ready to act fast - physically, emotionally, mentally, spiritually. Otherwise we strike out again and again. What we do daily, matters.

Are you going to sit back on your water float, and try to drink that glass of lemonade, blind to the oncoming monster of a wave? Or will you join me and many others, as we train ourselves to be awesome surfers on the waves churning in the great ocean of life? I know I have work to do. I plan to have fun doing the work. Preparing myself. I plan to go on this journey supporting and being supported with a community of like minded souls. This makes me smile.

Even if tomorrow, the world turns around, the worst is over, and we can all sit on our water lily water floats and sip lemonade, I will still have my dharma. All my efforts will still be needed and will still bear fruit. We might as well enjoy the journey together even if we don't know how long the ride will be. We can be working hard, overcoming challenges and be full of joy - joy, joy, joy, ever new joy!

Joy to you!

You can do this. We can do it together. I believe in you.

Your Calling

Have you ever reflected on your childhood dreams? Have you ever felt called to do something? Have you been given a calling and it has remained as a seed - as perhaps have your dreams, your larger aspirations, your dharma - your life's purpose?

When I had my own yoga studio The Marina Yoga and Health Center in San Francisco, I had students who were interested in learning yoga more in depth and even becoming yoga teachers. I would tell them to go where I went to learn - Ananda's Expanding Light Retreat Center. No matter how enticing I spoke of the experience, they didn't seem to want to take my advice to attend the training at the retreat center.

My students said "We want to learn from you!". I said, "Oh, you will learn so much more if you go to Ananda.". They replied "We are here. We don't want to go. We want to learn from you." Finally, I got the message! I began teaching my first yoga teacher training back in the 1980's.

Just like for so many years, I didn't tell anyone that I can read chakras. Just like I thought, preparing for times ahead would be done by others, I was slow to come around to the understanding that I am one of the ones to help others prepare, to be the best version of themselves. And help them to feel loved, supported and nurtured so that they can do the work that like you, they have been called to do. I moved from not only understanding, but fully realizing what I need to do. There is no turning back, there is only forward. Or if I stand still, like anyone else - we get knocked down by the ocean wave.

Sometimes pursuing or following your dharma can feel scary. You might feel like you are paving the way for things you have not seen or experienced and you don't know what is around the next corner. Often it will take you out of your comfort zone. And it's ok.

Maybe you are like one of my many clients, who need to feel validated and encouraged, to do what you know you should do, and have your calling clarified. They say after a chakra reading, how much lighter they feel, how encouraging it is for someone to see and understand them — and their situation, their challenges as well as their gifts. I see you. I believe in you.

I got to where I am today because I had help. Yes, I do a lot on my own as is also my nature. But I have teachers, mentors, coaches and wonderful colleagues. I also took some wrong turns, following advice from coaches who never took the time to understand who I really was and what I brought to the table from my life's experiences, talents and character.

I was in just such a program when I met Rafael, the Shaman who inspired this book series. We could see eye to eye and look beneath the surface and saw the seeds of pure potential in each other. Often we go down the wrong path because we need to meet someone, learn lessons and grow. Thus it was for me, for Steph the publisher, and some of the other authors in this series.

I was honored and blessed to be asked to lead the Ascension Ceremony for Rafael. I know that as a mature Shaman, Rafael is able to continue his important work that is his dharma, even as he is no longer in his body. Can you say the same for yourself?

I know that is a big metaphysical question. What I want to ask is, are you in a position to make a difference now, to follow your life's calling or are you still dreaming, maybe stuck, perhaps dabbling and playing small and safe? If you are, that's ok - for now. As time moves on though you will find that it's not actually the safe position you thought it was. Think, sneaker waves...

To play big, to do what you are truly meant to do, doesn't require a giant leap. In fact, the bigger your dream, your calling, your dharma, the smaller the steps you need to take. A big leap across a river will land you in the middle of the river, wet and sore from the fall. Why not look for the exposed rocks to take step by step to get you safely to the other side? Better yet, ask someone experienced, where is the bridge?

Moving forward can be and usually is scary, even if you are excited and willing. Taking the small steps on the rocks, can still land you in the water if you slip, though the fall won't be so hard. And truth be told, sometimes the bridge can be slippery too. That's where our daily habits, that help us to be more centered, calm, focused, strong, flexible and balanced come in to play. Having a personal guide helps too.

Imagine a big ship in the ocean. It is hundreds of miles away from it's destination. If that ship's GPS is off just by a degree or two, it will land way off of it's course. Likewise, it often only takes a small adjustment in the direction that you are headed, to get you on track to your destination. Small habits can yield big results.

Take the time now, to let go of your old ways that no longer serve you. Nurture yourself and be kind to yourself as you explore your new direction, your reset GPS, and prepare to move full speed ahead. And don't forget, a ship has a full crew. You don't have to do this alone.

Now is the time. Now is the time for you to step into your dharma, fulfill your dreams and be a force of light in this world. I see you. I believe in you. If you are reading these words I know there is something more for you to do. Something more for you to fulfill.

And what is the consequence for not doing more? You guessed it! The next wave will knock you down. Each wave is going to get bigger and harder. It will be a long time before the sea calms down and the waves once again become playful. And we can sit on the beach and drink lemonade.

There is a guided affirmation-experience that I find myself giving to my students and private clients more and more. It is the "You Are Loved" guided meditation (because it is really hard to do scary things by ourselves, especially feeling unloved or unsupported). The good news is that you don't have to do it alone!

You are loved,
nurtured,
cared for,
supported.
You are loved unconditionally.

Though we are each unique, we have our own dharma, path to walk, we can spend time walking together, being nurtured together, collaborating, co-creating and simply yet powerfully being a loving witness to each other's destiny. I want you to know that you are unconditionally loved. You are loved, supported, cared for and nurtured.

I wish you effortless ease as you open into the next level of financial abundance, feeling loved, supported and nurtured on life's journey - the journey of following your dharma.

Enjoy!

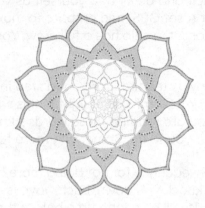

Everyone deserves Yoga Therapy that's done in a safe way, keeping in mind their unique life situation. That might be the trauma of being in prison or the complexities of being in a women's shelter. I think that yoga therapists are uniquely qualified to work with these populations.

~ Ann, C-IAYT

The Digital Revolution in the Age of Energy

Nicole DeAvilla,
E-RYT500, RPYT, RCYT, C-IAYT

The Rise of the Lotus Blossoms

Let's face it. We are in the mud at the bottom of a lake right now. Hopefully this book is nurturing you, as you dig your roots deep into the fertile soil. I encourage you to look up and see through the muddy water to the light shining on the lake's surface. That light, the fresh air, the peace of a lake full of a multitude of varied colored and shaped lotus blossoms living harmoniously together, is our future.

We're doing more than just imagining a future; we're actively inviting it into our present reality. Using our techniques of yoga we call upon the power of our minds to help shape our reality. The integration of ancient wisdom and modern technology will result in a new age in the annals of Yoga Therapy—a sacred future where lifestyle diseases become relics of the past, and holistic well-being becomes the norm. This is the Age of Energy, of Dwapara Yuga as the yogis call it.

When it comes to technology, I have always approached it with the thought of understanding how these tools can foster deeper human connections. With an early immersion into social media, I found a new way to offer the healing capabilities of Yoga Therapy, including the elements of community and connection. By harnessing this modern medium, I also had the privilege of supporting my fellow healers and authors, amplifying their messages of well-being and transformation to a wider audience. As we venture further into this fascinating crossroads of ancient practice and modern life rising from the mud and into the beautiful light of the day, transformation is truly limitless.

Two Sides of the Same Coin?

Yoga and technology might seem like strange bedfellows, but my personal journey showed me that they are more like two sides of the same coin—complementing rather than conflicting with each other.

While on the one side of the coin, AI algorithms analyze biometric data, testing scientific hypotheses at lightning speed either shedding light on a promising cure or proving futility so quickly, researchers are free to move onto the next one. This is one example of the Age of Energy as expressed in technological advances.

On the other side of the coin is a renewal and greater awareness of subtle energy. My ability to read a person's chakras, their inner energy field, to help facilitate their healing process and spiritual journey, will cease to be a strange anomaly and become commonplace. This is one example of the Age of Energy as expressed through the metaphysical.

I have pioneered and embraced technology over and over again. Yes, I am aware of and mostly avoid its pitfalls. I feel strongly that when harnessed by heart centered, compassionate human beings like you and me, we can help shape the future of AI and not be ruled by it. In fact as a yogi, a Yoga Therapist and conscious entrepreneur, I see it as my duty to not sit idly by and hope AI won't take over the world!

"The Minutes Are More Important Than the Years"
Parmahansa Yogananda

As we all embrace the positive uses of AI, time becomes more available for the personal connections that we have been losing through other forms of technology.

With the advent of AI now racing into nearly every aspect of our lives, human touch, eye contact, the human spark of connecting at a soul level, becomes more precious. Think of artificial intelligence as the benevolent force behind the scenes, tirelessly sifting through data, handling administrative tasks, automating repetitive work, and helping to plan a family vacation. This isn't just about efficiency; it's about reclaiming our most precious resource—time.

The ancient yogis taught us that time is an illusion, so why do we need more of it? Because we are still bound by it. Just as Yogananda said, if you can heal your broken bone by the power of your mind, then do so, otherwise have a doctor do it. Likewise, if you can live your life fully liberated of time, then do so. In the meantime, use your time wisely.

Though I have experienced first-hand, time standing still, time rushing forward and the feel of the past and the future merged into the present, it is not my constant reality. It is my practice. It is in the present moment that we are taught to live. In each present moment we can use this precious "extra time" wisely or fritter it away.

The road into this future of hope and possibility, of peace, connection and greater wellbeing, is bumpy and perhaps washed out in places! This calls for the greater application of our yogic tools to see us through with the fewest bumps and bruises as possible. I hope that you can see, that you can feel from the stories, examples and simple Yoga Therapy found in these pages, that yoga practices can see us through just about anything.

As Krishna says in the Bhagavad Gita, Even a little practice of this dharma (religious rite or righteous action) will save you from dire fear and colossal suffering.

Whereas yoga in popular culture has shed many of its more profound, deeper healing and higher consciousness elevating aspects, the Yoga Therapists of the world have been keeping its sacred essence intact. They know that to help people on an individual level it requires the entire yogic tool box; to meet people where they are, where they are going and honor what is unique and beautiful in each person.

Knowledge is Power

I believe knowledge is power. The sacred knowledge of ancient yoga is a powerful force. The understanding and knowledge of the workings of AI, is a powerful force. As a yogi, I have gone out of my way to learn as much as I can in this new frontier of AI and bring it back to you. Just as I translate the Sanskrit into modern language to make yoga useful and accessible in our modern age, I am here to translate the basics of AI, so that you will find it not a burden or something to fear. Rather it can become a new tool in our toolbox.

In essence, we are the architects of a new world, one that holds the promise of holistic success and well-being for all, irrespective of their background. The best of both worlds is not just an idyllic dream; it's a future we can, and must, create. So, let's rise and beckon our lotus buds into full bloom, use the gift of these magnificent toolboxes, and build a sacred future that will stand as a testament to human innovation and compassion. Are you ready to join this incredible journey?

In Full Bloom

Let's look beyond the horizon together. This is not just my story; it's our story. It's a narrative that belongs to anyone willing to venture into the extraordinary landscape of possibilities. I invite you to embrace both the promises of ancient sacred yoga and a future where we all live peacefully in the same multi-colored, varied lotus pond of this world. Together, we can create a future that's not only extraordinary but also deeply rooted in authenticity and wisdom. Now's the time.

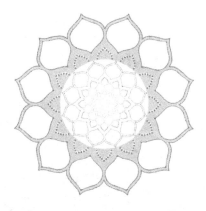

There is a Sanskrit saying that means, "Practice yoga daily and stay disease free." It is preventive medicine.

~Dillip, C-IAYT

A Note from the Publisher

Steph Ritz with RitzBooks.com

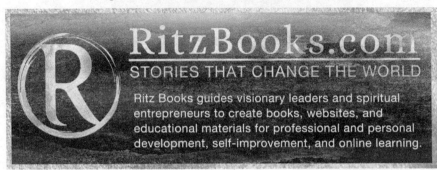

Steph's Sacred Writing Experiences
to Inspire Wisdom from Within

Ritz Books brings together authors and artists from around the world to offer you their healing magic. I hope you enjoyed these life-altering messages that celebrate individual differences, who we are at the core, and offers glimpses into our shared humanity.

It is my wish that these books reveal the potential that lies within your heart, uncover possibilities within yourself, and guide you to embrace ultimately creating individual and global transformation. More than that, I wish to offer you a glimpse into the healing magic you have to offer the world.

What you are inspired to write is meant to be shared - not sit inside of you. Please, don't take what lives inside of you to your grave, don't take tomorrow for granted...

Before departing this life, please share your insights, beliefs, and experiences with the world. Take a moment to listen to the voice of your heart and set your wishes sailing in the sky. It's time to leave your legacy.

Meet Steph Ritz

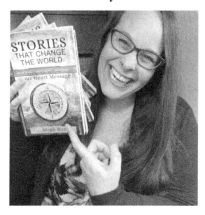

Steph Ritz is the publisher, graphic designer, coach and editor of this book. With dozens of international bestselling books, she is a world-renowned writer, web designer, and photographer. Steph combines cutting-edge writing techniques, deep connection, and taking effective action to create stories that change the world.

Hybrid Publishing with Ritz Books under the imprint "Ritz Books" yet managed from your Amazon account, so you get 100% of the royalties. Collaboration books donate their royalties to non-profits and scholarship funds. Both hybrid publishing and collaborative books include ghostwriting, editing, cover design, and layout.

"Steph's marketing is like the Slow Food movement. It's not as fast and convenient as traditional marketing, but it creates a higher quality result without the indigestion! Steph Ritz helped me understand what it takes so people hear me and see me as an expert. She helped me learn to express myself with clarity and purpose – which led to integrated packages for my coaching clients and rebranding my 2 Minute Yoga website."
~ Nicole DeAvilla

Ritz Books Authors

Adhana McCarthy, Illinois

Agnes Barna, Sydney, Australia

Angela Heart, California

Annie B. Kay, Massachusetts

Banton Dyer, Texas

Cristina Laskar, California

Cynthia "Oya Gbemi" Barnes, Florida

Dara Bayer, Massachusetts

Debbie Howard, Texas & Japan

Etoke "Fuatabong Lekeanju" Atabong, Maryland & Cameroon, Africa

Glenys Brown, Perth, Australia

Grace Lawrence, Oregon

Hasti Fashandi, California

Ilene Cohen, California

Jay Rooke, California

Jenny McFadden, Sydney, Australia

Jermaine "Spirit Buffalo" Reeves, Kentucky

Julia Lewis, Virginia

Kimberly "Omiseun" Early, Washington

LaVerne "Nzinga" Gyant, Illinois

Lee Blackwell, Lake Macquarie, Australia

Lisa "AyoDeji" Allen, Pennsylvania

Lorna Patten, Cammeray, Australia

Louise Elliott, Canberra Australia

Makhosi Yeye Gogo Nana Omari, Maryland

Mariyamah "OloMidara" Hill-Sanna, Ohio & Ghana, Africa

Marshall "OmiTosin" Henderson Jr., Tennessee

Mesfen Manna, Kentucky

Michelle Bee, California

Nashid "Koleoso" Fakhrid-Deen (1949-2020)

Nicole DeAvilla, California

Pat Southern-Pearce, Manchester, United Kingdom

Phyllis Douglass (Vox Angelus), California

Preeti Gupta, Kentucky & New Delhi, India

Radcliffe Johnson, California

Ralph Stevenson, Pennsylvania

Regina "Abegunde" Harris, Kentucky

Robin "Osunnike" Scott-Manna, Kentucky

Robin Daw, California

Roza Bann, Sydney, Australia

Sebastian Laskar, California

Sorcha Fraser-Swatton, Mudgee, Australia

Steph Ritz, California

Tomas Reyes, California & Columbia, South America

Vivian Geffen, Arizona

When tested, we are all stronger than we imagined, smarter than we give ourselves credit for, and have the resiliency of a dandelion... for when the light calls, we will rise again.

~ Steph Ritz

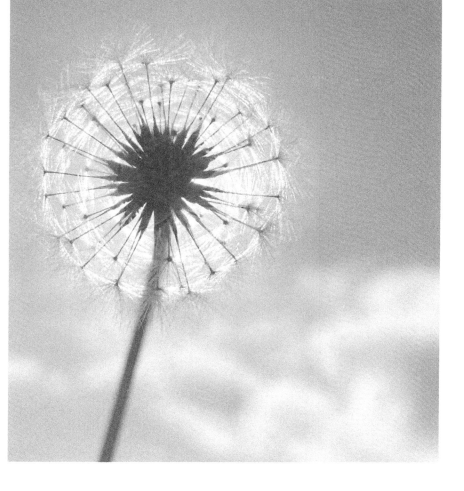